ZOMBIES

UNIVERSITY PRESS OF FLORIDA

Florida A&M University, Tallahassee
Florida Atlantic University, Boca Raton
Florida Gulf Coast University, Ft. Myers
Florida International University, Miami
Florida State University, Tallahassee
New College of Florida, Sarasota
University of Central Florida, Orlando
University of Florida, Gainesville
University of North Florida, Jacksonville
University of South Florida, Tampa
University of West Florida, Pensacola

BY THE SAME AUTHOR

Zombis: Enquête sur les morts-vivants, Tallandier, 2015

Quand la science explore l'histoire, in collaboration with David Alliot, Paris, Tallandier, 2014.

(ed.) *Seine de crimes*, Paris, Le Rocher, 2014.

(ed.) *Actes du 4ᵉ colloque international de pathographie* (Saint-Jean-de-Côle, May 2011), in collaboration with D. Gourevitch, Paris, De Boccard, *Pathographie* 9, 2013.

Henri IV, l'énigme du roi sans tête, in collaboration with S. Gabet, Paris, Vuibert, 2013.

Paris au scalpel: Itinéraires secrets d'un médecin légiste, Paris, Le Rocher, 2012.

Autopsie de l'art premier, Paris, Le Rocher, 2012.

Les secrets des grands crimes de l'histoire, Paris, Vuibert, 2012.

(ed.) *Le miroir du temps: Les momies de Randazzo (XVIIᵉ–XIXᵉ siècle)*, in collaboration with L. Lo Gerfo, Paris, De Boccard, *Pathographie* 7, 2011.

(ed.) *Le roman des morts secrètes de l'histoire*, Paris, Le Rocher, 2011.

(ed.) *Actes du 3ᵉ colloque international de pathographie* (Bourges, April 2009), Paris, De Boccard, *Pathographie* 6, 2011.

(ed.) *Actes du 2ᵉ colloque international de pathographie* (Loches, April 2007), Paris, De Boccard, *Pathographie* 4, 2009.

Male mort: Morts violentes dans l'Antiquité, Paris, Fayard, 2009.

Les jeunes filles et la mort: Catalogue de l'exposition, Bourges, Les 1000 univers, 2009.

Maladies humaines, thérapies divines: Analyse épigraphique et paléopathologique de textes de guérison grecs, in collaboration with C. Prêtre, Lille, PUS, 2009.

(ed.) *Ostéo-archéologie et techniques médico-légales*, Paris, De Boccard, *Pathographie* 2, 2008.

Les monstres humains dans l'Antiquité: Analyse paléopathologique, Paris, Fayard, 2008.

(ed.) *Actes du 1ᵉʳ colloque international de pathographie* (Loches, April 2005), Paris, De Boccard, *Pathographie* 1, 2007.

Médecin des morts: Récits de paléopathologie, Paris, Fayard, 2006; *Pluriel*, 2014.

The first problem is to know when the dead are truly dead.

DR. NATHAN KLINE

(quoted in *The Serpent and the Rainbow* by Wade Davis)

CONTENTS

AUTHOR'S PREFACE TO THE ENGLISH EDITION

The Republic of Haiti, one of the oldest in the world, amasses frequent natural disasters within its territory, including earthquakes, cholera epidemics, and very recently, a devastating hurricane. With each calamity, neo-Protestant churches that proliferate within the territory present magical-religious explanations. These include a curse cast upon the island by the Gods of the Vodou pantheon or the wrath of the Christian God angered by the presence of devil worshippers on the island (in other words, Vodouists). No matter what the explanation might be, it is a clash of civilizations exacerbated in these times of crisis that natural disasters and their bloodshed represent.

The other result of these large-scale human dramas is the rampant appearance of individuals who are socially considered to be zombies in the weeks or months that follow these crises.

This volume explains both the entire current situation and the appropriateness to carry out an anthropological investigation in Haiti in order to better understand this phenomenon and to assess the very polymorphic character of it. There is not one "zombie" (least of all the zombie from the film industry, which is a very recent creation that is "distorted" from the original myth), but many zombies whose meaning and creative concepts vary depending on need.

The zombie is a stopgap of our imagination, of lonely families, or even of simple justice. But zombies are most definitely present. They are tangible, real fantasies. And they are not about to disappear.

Since the publication of the first edition (in French) of this book, other zombies have been reported on the island, making the headlines of local newspapers and feeding this fascination with death and the occult. Max Beauvoir, the *ati*, has passed away, or rather, his soul has returned to

Africa, to the land of the ancestors. But his soul continues to bring beneficial help to his heirs, starting with *mambo* Mireille. Life goes on. Spells persist. There is not yet any law to protect zombies who have escaped the clutches of their creators (the *bokors*), but the plan is advancing. The health and economic crisis to come should accelerate things.

This book is a dive into the world of Haitian zombies with a dual emphasis in medicine and anthropology. In order to successfully complete this research, it was necessary to attend rituals and to visit cemeteries under the cloak of night. It was necessary to collect Vodou dolls and, once back in Europe, to examine them by X-ray. It was necessary to drink and to dance. It was necessary to see hermetic symbols sketched on the ground that were aimed at *loas*. It was necessary to visit the high security areas of psychiatric hospitals and the Court in Port-au-Prince. It was necessary to make atoning sacrifices in order to secure the word of men, etc. This is indeed the price to pay to reveal a few of the scientific mysteries surrounding zombies.

TRANSLATOR'S NOTE

I would like to thank the following people for their helpful advice and suggestions at the various stages of the preparation of this translation: Benjamin Hebblethwaite, associate professor in Haitian Creole, Haitian and Francophone studies, for having recommended me as the translator of this study and for his offer to explain certain Creole terminology;[1] Jennifer Rathbun, professor of Spanish and chair of the Department of Foreign Languages at Ashland University, who contributed invaluable advice at the initial phases of this translation; and, finally, the author, Philippe Charlier, who kindly answered my request for clarification and explanations. I would be remiss if I did not express my gratitude to my wife and our four children, Geneviève, Madeleine, Catherine and RJ, who always add to my work in some way and who are always impacted by the time required to complete projects such as this one. Thank you.

This translation attempts to remain as faithful as possible to the original author's language, sentence structure, registers, and the overall texture of the source text. There is arguably some variation in English/Creole/French terminology as well as in the spelling of Caribbean words. At times, I have kept the original French/Creole words, italicized, and sometimes I have used an English equivalent. A glossary has been included to help with terminology that might be unfamiliar to the reader. Philippe Charlier has a writing style that is all his own. His sentence structure—syntax and punctuation—is fluid. He also uses a range of voices. Sometimes, he uses the voice of a storyteller. On other occasions, he uses the voice of a trained physician. When appropriate, I have followed the author's lead and maintained the voice of that of a forensic pathologist conducting an anthropological investigation. From the beginning of the text, I made difficult choices with regard to adapting his vocabulary and style to the English language.

The original title of the text, *Zombis: Enquête anthropologique sur les morts-vivants*, presented a true translation aporia. In English, the word *enquête* has several possible translations (survey; investigation; inquiry; questionnaire; study; inquest; probe; examination; poll; quest), several of which initially appear suitable to describe Charlier's work. After eliminating any options that did not fully describe my understanding of this text, I narrowed the list of possibilities to two terms: inquiry and investigation. Merriam Webster's Dictionary defines "inquiry" as: 1. "a request for information; 2. an official effort to collect and examine information about something; 3. the act of asking questions in order to gather or collect information." In comparison, Webster's defines "investigation" as: 1. "to try to find out the facts about (something, such as a crime or an accident) in order to learn how it happened, who did it, etc.; 2. to try to get information about (someone who may have done something illegal)." At first blush, it appears that we could use either word to describe the study that Charlier has fashioned. A quick glance at the etymologies of the verbs "to inquire" and "to investigate," however, reveals a thought-provoking difference in perspective underscored by the translator's lexical choice. Merriam Webster's Dictionary states that "to inquire" comes from the Middle English verb "*enquiren,* from Anglo-French *enquerre,* from Vulgar Latin **inquaerere,* alteration of Latin *inquirere,* from *in-* + *quaerere* to seek" (13th century). The etymology of "to investigate," in contrast, is from the "Latin *investigatus,* past participle of *investigare* to track, investigate, from *in-* + *vestigium* footprint, track (First Known Use: circa 1510)." Therefore, the choice of whether to translate the title of Charlier's text as *An Anthropological Inquiry on the Living Dead* or *An Anthropological Investigation of the Living Dead* ultimately comes down to whether or not the translator—or the reader, for that matter—sees the author's purpose in developing this study as a quest for information or as a footprint or track. In my reading of this text, I see Philippe Charlier first and foremost as a scientist tracing a pathway ["footprint" or "track" (investigation)] toward an understanding of how zombification functions in modern-day Haiti. Alain Froment's comments in the Postface support my interpretation.

It is for this reason that I have chosen to interpret Charlier's text as an "investigation."

In the course of translating this text, several additional lexical items presented thought-provoking challenges, including the author's repeated use of the nouns "fantasme" and "imaginaire." We can translate "fantasme" in English as "fantasy," "dream," "phantasm," or "delusion." In most contexts presented within this text, "fantasy" is the most reasonable choice. The author's use of the word "imaginaire," which we might commonly translate as either "imagination" or "fantasy," however, relates more closely to the American-English notion of "mind" or "mindset" in the sense of a "way of thinking" or a "perspective" rather than an "imagination" or a "fantasy." What emerges in this text is both a flexibility and a fluidity in the way in which Charlier expresses these seemingly complementary nouns. Contrastingly, although Charlier is a trained medical doctor, his use of the word "cadavre" almost always means "corpse" in the sense of a dead body that one might see after the process of zombification is complete, rather than "cadaver" in the medical sense of the term. Furthermore, in order to minimize negative connotations of the word "voodoo," throughout this translation I have chosen to use the spelling "Vodou" rather than the more common "voodoo." Individuals who study the Vodou religion in the Americas prefer this particular spelling.

Charlier's use of the words "tombe" and "tombeau" also created an interesting situation. In English, "tombe" can mean either "grave" or "tomb." We could translate the French word "tombeau" in similar fashion. For most American-English speakers, however, the words "grave" and "tomb" are not completely interchangeable. The word "grave" functions in a very basic sense to describe a burial place. In contrast, the word "tomb" can refer to a building or chamber that is either above or below the ground in which a dead body is kept, thus flooding the mind with images such as King Tut's tomb or Jesus's "tomb." For the purposes of this translation, I have made a concerted effort to respect the original flavor of Charlier's words while at the same time attempting to avoid any inaccurate connotations.

It is also important to mention that the term "médecin légiste" used in Charlier's text has three possible English translations: forensic pathologist, medical examiner, and coroner. These three professions are not completely synonymous. A forensic pathologist is a medical professional who specializes in determining the cause of death. He or she is a medical doctor who has completed training in anatomical pathology and who has sub-specialized in forensic pathology. A forensic pathologist is not necessarily an appointed public officer. A medical examiner, in contrast, is an appointed public officer with duties similar to those of a coroner but who is required to have specific medical training (as in pathology) and is qualified to conduct medical examinations and autopsies. A coroner, in comparison, is an elected public officer who is normally not required to have specific medical qualifications and whose main responsibility is to investigate the cause of any death when there is reason to suspect that the death is not the result of natural causes. In this translation, I have chosen the English-language term that is most suitable to the given context.

Finally, in the course of completing this translation, my most interesting translation challenge concerned how to translate Charlier's frequent use of the word "cercueil," translated in English as either "coffin" or "casket." To many native English speakers, these two words initially appear to be interchangeable. Closer examination, however, reveals that although coffins and caskets have the same function, they differ essentially on their respective designs. Coffins are typically wide at the shoulders and tapered at the head and foot with a cover that extends the entire length of the frame. Caskets, in contrast, are rectangular in shape, are typically constructed of quality woods or metals, and feature higher standards of craftsmanship. Caskets also typically include a cover that opens halfway, thus allowing the lower extremities of the deceased individual's body to remain concealed. Until the fourteenth chapter of his text, the word "cercueil" had held little distinctive descriptive value to me. It was not until the author mentioned that these "cercueils" are "wooden and metal caskets, mostly American imports (Batesville, Indiana) . . . all padded with foam cushions and . . . covered in spotless white polyester" (152) that my own experience and a translator revealed a fuller context to me.

In the summer of 1998, as part of the background to inform a translation project that I had been hired to prepare on the subject of burial practices in France, I was flown to Indianapolis, Indiana, and driven to

Batesville to participate in a guided tour of the Batesville Casket Company's manufacturing facilities. There, I learned both about U.S. burial practices directly from the largest casket manufacturer in the United States and how these burial customs compared with those in other parts of the world. Through safety goggles, I saw assembly line workers producing a range of both wooden and metal caskets. My tour concluded with a visit to a "Showroom" displaying a variety of caskets ranging from Batesville's least expensive bronze, copper, oak, and pine caskets to the top-of-the-line President® model made of exquisite mahogany. Many Batesville hardwood caskets feature a MemorySafe® drawer in which loved ones can place objects that are important to the departed individual. Hence, as a result of my visit to the Batesville Casket Company's manufacturing facilities and the knowledge that I acquired there nearly two decades ago, I chose to use the word "casket" almost exclusively when describing the "cercueils" used in Haiti. Given Charlier's specific reference to Batesville, Indiana and the understanding that this manufacturer produces a wide range of caskets from the very inexpensive to the most luxurious, this lexical choice is reasonable. In situations in which Charlier uses "cercueil" to refer to its use in Europe, however, I employ the word "coffin" to indicate this particular distinction. Such situations are nonetheless infrequent within the present study.

It is my hope that the English translation of Philippe Charlier's text entitled *Zombis: Enquête anthropologique sur les morts-vivants* will convey to Anglophone readers both the depth of his understanding of the zombie phenomenon within Haiti at the same time that it deconstructs the many misunderstandings surrounding the zombie and the Vodou religion as a whole, particularly within the United States.

Note

1. For a detailed dictionary of Vodou terms, see Hebblethwaite's text entitled *Vodou Songs in Haitian Creole and English* (Philadelphia: Temple University Press, 2012).

ZOMBIES

CHAPTER 1

ZOMBIE

What Are We Talking About?

For nearly a century, zombies have served as an archetype of the fear of the return of the dead. They represent as much the incarnation of *post mortem* physical alterations as the fear of the misdiagnosis of death (a false declaration of death with an unjustified burial).

In the Western mindset, they have served as an outlet for the harshest of anxieties and fantasies, and sometimes also the most harebrained. First limited to the geographic area of the Caribbean, zombies quickly become a cut-and-paste of the vampire myth, and spread widely throughout the continent of North America. This fact is evidenced by the abundance of films and television series featuring the phenomenon of zombies, especially from the American film industry, including *I Walked with a Zombie* (Jacques Tourneur, 1943), *Night of the Living Dead* (George A. Romero, 1968), which constructs itself as a parable of the evils of America, the saga *Resident Evil*, and the television series *The Walking Dead* (five seasons in all, and a worldwide success), etc.

But these monstrous beings, in fact, have nothing to do with the real zombie that comes from Haitian Vodou. If anything, they represent a sort of realization of the medieval myth of the decayed ghost (the "putrid revenant"). These are living-dead that come out of the Earth, continue their decomposition above ground, and change humans into zombies through

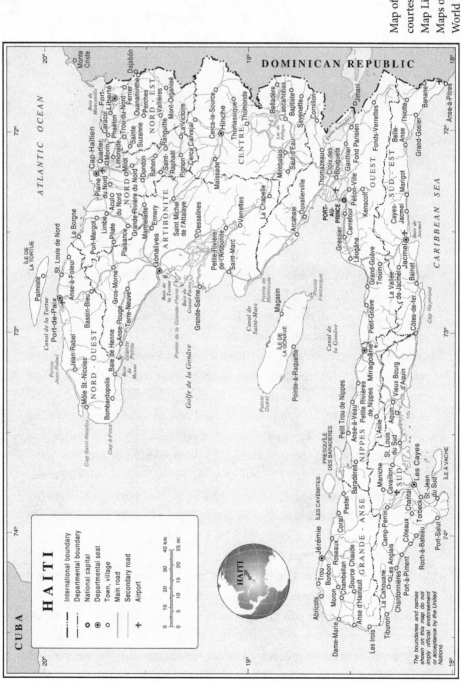

Map of Haiti, courtesy of Map Library/ Maps of the World

a bite or simple contact. In order to survive, they sometimes must eat brains and suck blood. It is as if zombification were a communicable disease, a type of modern allegory for the ancestral fear of the Plague.

The term zombie takes on three meanings that are quite similar to each other. The first, which is no longer accepted, refers to children who died without being baptized whose souls have been captured in order to bring good luck.[1] The second corresponds to a ghostly spirit which, flying away from the corpse at the moment of death, moves around detached from the body like a wandering soul. It can appear either in human form or it can be without a specific form, like a moving cloud. Finally, the last type—and the most commonly accepted—is the individual to whom a poison was given that put him in a cataleptic state. They pass him off as dead, and then he is buried before being exhumed from the cemetery two or three days later in order to turn him into a zombie.

With a perspective that is both forensic and anthropological, I found it interesting to go back to the source. Why does Haiti, this island in the Caribbean, inscribe itself within the collective imagination as the historical land of zombies? To what do zombies correspond? Can they be summed up as the simple victims of an animal poison? Are they nothing but a literary creation picked up by the film industry? Do they play a social, moral, or political role? In the 1980s, the work of Wade Davis, a North American ethnobotanist, cleared the way for this subject by identifying a molecule implicated in zombification. But is this research continuing to move forward? Will the medical and scientific study of new cases of zombies enable us to know more about the process of their "creation"?

I thus left to conduct an anthropological investigation of the traces of these beings who are between two worlds. It is an anthropological investigation between life and death.

CHAPTER 2

WHITE ZOMBIE

The Air Caraïbes aircraft has been in flight for several hours and must set itself roughly vertical to the Azores. In the darkness, the passengers sleep peacefully. Some snore while sleeping off their little bottles of coconut punch. Others try their luck with the flight attendants. I make the most of the situation by turning on my computer to watch the film *White Zombie* for the one hundredth time. It is an old black-and-white film (1932) that marks one of the first appearances of Bela Lugosi.

This film—the first cinematographic work to dramatize zombies—opens with a horse-drawn carriage on a country road winding through the middle of a sugarcane field at night. The carriage is transporting two Westerners who have just landed at Port-au-Prince. On the road, they stumble across a funeral ceremony. Peasants, weeping, are burying one of their own in the very middle of the road.

"We'd call it a burial. . . .

—On the road? . . . What's going on?

—It's a funeral, Miss. They fear grave robbers, so they dig graves in the middle of the road where there is a lot of traffic . . . ," the coach driver explains (he is a Haitian with a strong Creole accent).

Emerging at that moment from a cemetery and the adjoining plantations are men dressed in rags with a glassy look and a rolling gait. Moving at breakneck speed, the horse-drawn carriage begins to flee the arrival of the zombies.

"You could have killed us driving at such speeds!

—Worse, Sir, we could have been captured!

—By whom? The men whom we ran into?

—They aren't men, sir. They're dead bodies. . . . Zombies. Living-dead. Corpses stolen from graves and made to work in the sugar mills and the fields at night."

CHAPTER 3

LAËNNEC HURBON

The exit from the airport is challenging. One must make one's way through the crowd of families that have come to wait for their relatives to disembark from the airplane. The vans of peacekeepers bearing the UN emblem park a few meters from the tarmac. Sub-machine guns are clearly visible. Outside, the air smells like Africa more than it does the Caribbean. It is a familiar scent like that of Cotonou, Lomé, or Lagos. The tone is set.

The car rolls quickly on the potholed roadways towards the periphery of Port-au-Prince. On the sidewalks, mobile vendors and tiny bungalows run alongside and resemble each other for several kilometers. *Dieu seul maître boutique* displays pyramids of Prestige (the local beer), *Soeur de Marie-Joseph rechaj* offers a selection of cellphone chargers, *La Trinité computer services, Ave Maria restaurant-bar, Christ matériaux de construction* (construction materials), *Avec Jésus dépôt de ciment* (cement depot), *Grâce divine quincaillerie* (hardware store), *Père éternel loto* (lottery), *Tout à Jésus pharmacie* (pharmacy), *La Nativité studio beauté* (beauty salon), colorful posters of evening concerts (Boukman, Eksperyans . . . Alfazombie!), religious establishments bearing bold names ("Tabernacle of the Evangelical Crusade"), etc.

On the rear bench seat of the car lies a copy of *Nouvelliste* (one of the daily newspapers of the Republic of Haiti). A large headline regarding "chèques zombis" sprawls across the front page—in other words, these are rubber checks. The concept of the zombie has truly entered into even the slightest of Haitian comings and goings. At the end of an hour, half asleep, I arrive at the home of Laënnec Hurbon, sociologist and research director at the CNRS (National Center for Scientific Research). Three art books on Haitian Vodou are placed on the living room coffee table. One of them, signed by Cristina García Rodero, is impressive.[1] The cover photo, in black and white, features a young disciple of the Vodou religion, dressed only in a dark loincloth, who is submerged in a lake of mud (called a *bain de chance*). With sluggishness and sensuality, the disciple turns around towards the goat kid that he is carrying on his shoulders and that he will soon sacrifice. It is a haunting and fascinating image.

From the very beginning of our conversation, Laënnec Hurbon asks me to put a little distance between myself and zombies. This man has studied what Haitian society is going through in this day and age enough to understand that this narrow connection between local inhabitants and the dead almost constitutes a friendship. Here, we are not trying to find out whether or not zombies exist. In the religious life of Haitians, the zombie is important, and they find a space within that life both to play with and to cheat death, to avoid it. The trauma of the slave trade has played a significant role in this phenomenon.

Does death bring about fascination? Is it feared? Is there an every-dayness about death? On the edge of the road, the Pharmacie Déliver-ance has painted a Bible verse on its front window: "It is good to wait quietly for the salvation of the LORD" (*Lamentations* 3:26). This is very reassuring. On the road between the airport in Port-au-Prince and the city center, I counted nearly one hundred private funeral homes, includ-ing *Mille souvenirs salon funéraire* (funeral parlor); *Jackson Jeanty salon funéraire* (funeral parlor), *morgue privée* (private morgue); *Saint-Clair maison funéraire* (funeral home), *assurance de décès* (life insurance), *gerbes de fleurs et couronnes* (flowers); *Fils de Dieu, entreprise funéraire* (funeral home); *Entreprise funéraire Bonne entente* (funeral home), etc., as if the dead were a part of daily life in the same way as the living, in nearly equal parts, and sometimes even in a dominant way. Indeed, some Haitians can spend their lives preparing their graves and their funerals. Here, dying is something that happens in stages. Once a person has died, he or she goes on a new pilgrimage that must lead, in turn, to becoming a guardian god for the community, the village, or the family. The individual must prevent his soul from wandering, and thus, captured by anyone, stop his soul from being misused, particularly within a context of sorcery. There is nothing worse than these wandering souls that drag their lot through sordid alleys or along major highways. For a Haitian, it is unbearable to think about such a future. Therefore, one must succeed in one's death.

This "success" is obtained through rituals that expect the dead individual to distance himself from the community because his presence causes confusion and creates general disarray. This disarray manifests itself both within the environment and in nature. This is clearly demonstrated by asking certain Haitians what takes place at the moment of death. They answer, "There is a star that disappears," "A meteor has crossed the sky to carry away his soul," etc. In other words, nature itself enters into the disarray process that death represents. Here, we encounter the theory of the microcosm/macrocosm (what happens here on Earth is only the shadow of what happens up there in the sky. Humans are only "the smallness of a greatness elsewhere").

There is something poetic about death. Haitian society does not turn the deceased person into either an object or someone who is disconnected from the world of the living. Beginning with this idea, a permanent back-and-forth is established between life and death. Moreover, the ritual of the *guédés* (spirits of the deceased) is one of the most important in Haiti. The individual who is possessed by a *guédé* says things that refer to death, of course, but that also discuss sexuality (hence, life), thus fluctuating periodically between Eros and Thanatos. This plethora of sexual expressions represents a type of embellishment of life.

The dead individual is not seen as something impure, but rather as something that challenges the system itself. All funeral rituals will have the goal of separating what is living from what is dead to assure the final departure of the dead from the community of the living, the deceased individual being considered potentially dangerous since he challenges the established order. It is only *a posteriori*—during the course of a reintegration ritual of the dead with the community—that the deceased can become a potential protector. Meanwhile, magical practices are designed to keep the deceased from returning to his home to spread disorder there. For example, in the countryside, the deceased cannot be driven to the cemetery without precautions. The pallbearers must appear to be on the wrong path so that the departed will not be able to find the road that would lead him back home.[2]

The individual is still connected to a community. Everything that has to do with death must be understood, coded, ritualized, and symbolized. More than a way of organizing chaos, it is a way to keep chaos from existing. In Haiti, there are funeral washing practices imported from Black Africa. There are "bathers of the dead" whose role is to prepare the deceased for the journey that begins at the final sigh. Because for Haitians, true life begins at the moment of death. Subsequently, this fateful moment brings together a large number of activities so that the deceased departs *condicio sine qua non* ("a condition without which it could not be") so that he might render a service to the living. For Vodouists, it is necessary to remove the protective force from the dead that they had during their life. The *déssouné* (or *dissouni*) is a ritual that thus consists of removing the *loa* to which they have been consecrated and which is still attached to their head. This is not a desecration, but rather a liberation. The *loa* is physically and intrinsically attached to the individual, and when the *loa* leaves the earthly body, the deceased can move and get up. In many morgues, one finds deceased individuals who are seated on the ground, even though they were brought in on stretchers. Some even resume their positions later. There are many stories about the dead in Haiti. "That happens," they say about this subject, with hardly any surprise.

The Republic of Haiti is at the convergence of three main cultures: Black African, Caribbean, and French. In these mixed beliefs about death and the destination of the dead, where does the zombie fit in?

The diverse testimonies that I successfully obtained from *houngans* or undertakers more-or-less describe the process. In Haiti, the deceased person is buried within 24 hours after death. In the event of zombification, in order to shorten this amount of time, the *bokor* (a Vodou priest practicing evil magic) must spread a vile-smelling liquid (emanating from a corpse in an advanced state of decomposition) around the house in order to pretend that there is an urgency to carrying out the burial. To lure the deceased out of his grave, the *bokor* or his aides use one of the victim's spiritual elements that they had previously kept and stored in a bottle (the *ti-bon-anj*) to turn him into a zombie. The *bokor* places himself at the foot of the grave with the bottle and makes the individual rise up. Attracted by its "soul fragment," the body will be removed from the tomb. Unable to leave alone, the deceased is exhumed by the *bokor*'s aides, the *loups-garous* (usually masons from the cemetery or individuals who bathe the dead, or even grave diggers) who shatter the masonry of the tomb, made of thin mortar—that is, with very little cement. Next, they take hold of the casket that they position headfirst in order to rush blood into the head of the "deceased." They bring out the body and rub it vigorously to relax the muscles and stimulate circulation. Finally, in order to finish awakening him completely, the *loups-garous* either make the individual swallow a potion made of *concombre zombi* leaves soaked in clarion (a strong alcohol) or they make him breathe the smoke of the same leaves that they burn at his feet. Next, they spray the zombie with icy water to finish awakening his senses, then violent lashes are administered to him with a whip to stimulate his nervous, peripheral, sensitive, and motor systems (and particularly to enable him to walk again in an effective way). They close his jaws with a strip of cloth to prevent him from screaming. Then, a *condeur* (or *conducteur*) wraps him up in a cloth shroud (so that he is not recognized by the nighttime wanderers who might run into the strange convoy) and he puts a rope around his waist to adjust the cloth better so as not to impede his ability to walk. Then, the *condeur* leads him to the *bokor*'s home. The *condeur* holds on to the other end of the rope. Sometimes the zombie's two arms are fastened at his back, sometimes his two thumbs are tied in front of him to unbalance him in the event that he attempts to run away (wrists or thumbs thus tied, he would fall immediately and would be very easy to catch).

From this moment, the zombie is remotely operated by this bottle filled with *ti-bon-anj* (the image of a remote control was used by Laënnec Hurbon). The *bokor* leads him either to the left or to the right in the simplest way. The use of *concombre zombi* (*Datura stramonium*, for some,

Momordica elaterum, for others) while removing the zombie from the gravesite and its possible repeated administration throughout the period of bondage could produce a state of extreme psychological passivity within the individual.[3]

The zombie represents the ideal of the individual who is enslaved to others. He places himself in the service of whoever ordered the act of zombification, a sort de punishment that is perhaps worse than death itself, as it is generally dictated by revenge and vengeance. The zombie will be put to work in a sugar cane field, or, because he is frightening, he will serve as the protector of a house (to monitor the walls or the people who live there). In any case, he toils. But he must not be given just any food. He must have his meals served on banana leaves (like the former slaves of Saint-Domingue). He must not function entirely as a human (he is almost human, but not quite). He is prohibited from having any alcohol and any substance that could awaken him. Salt is also forbidden (in magic, salt being considered the food of life? Or is it to leave the zombie in a chronic state of hyponatremia?).

Within this connotation of zombification, there are elements that spotlight fact and others that reveal fantasy and the symbolic (which is problematic to many researchers who come to Haiti to study the zombie, but without knowing that this term includes two very different concepts both socially and spiritually). The obsession of some researchers with toxic zombifying substances (mainly due to the influence of the work of ethnobotanist Wade Davis in the 1980s) sometimes makes them forget the other more social or religious aspects of the zombie. Of course, in a few fish, toads, leaves, etc., there are found products capable of reducing the vital capabilities of certain individuals, of putting them in a catatonic state, and even of giving them the appearance of death. But that is not all that there is to it. The phenomenon of zombies is much more complex.

Would it not be possible to add to these two a third type of zombie, one of a psychiatric nature—that is to say, subjects who, without having taken any particular drug and without being ghosts in the magical-religious sense, are in an abnormal state and give the impression of "living dead" (a type of necromimia)? The differential diagnosis of toxic zombification could, in effect, consist of the existence of a psychiatric illness that would remove the sociable character of the individual. We think mainly of schizophrenia (personality doubling), but we must not neglect another pathological entity: Cotard's disease. French neurologist Jules Cotard described this disease in 1880. A female patient had come to consult him, convinced that she had neither brain, nor nerves, nor chest, nor stomach, nor intestines, and considering herself nor more than a body in decomposition. She believed neither in God nor in Satan, and—according to her— had neither a soul nor any need to eat (she died shortly afterwards from cachexia).[4] Other cases have since been described within medical literature, some of them pre-dating Cotard's publication: an old woman, victim of an attack in 1788, who, during her convalescence, asked her daughters to dress her in a shroud and place her in a coffin because she was convinced that she was dead (she survived for three months in this state);[5] a pregnant woman, 28 years of age, convinced that her liver was in the process of rotting, and that her heart was missing; a man (Graham Harrison)[6] who made a suicide attempt by electrocution in a bathtub, then awoke in the hospital convinced that he was in a brain-dead state (his brain having been "fried" during the incident), and from then on spent his days frequenting cemeteries "in order to get closer to death."

For Laënnec Hurbon, this psychiatric view is too Western, and this third type of zombie matches the social zombie to a great extent(for whom toxic substances do not systematically interfere): the individual himself, in fact, recounts the story of his own zombification, whether it was a fantasy (caused by the individual himself) or caused by another person. The zombie is already structured by society. The subject enters the established structure and has almost no choice regarding symptoms or grievances. He identifies himself with a pre-existing zombie category, with all of its mythological cavalcade. He develops this group of clinical symptoms towards those who approach him, whether they are a psychiatrist, a priest, his family, or a stranger. Thus, there is no real psychological disorder, but rather a complete adherence to the magical-religious beliefs of zombification, or, at minimum, to their Haitian social form. In sum, this view draws closer to the traditional African concept that no death or illness is natural, but is always caused by others, and that no psychiatric illness exists, but only magical and spiritual possession.

For this to become possible, a dual problem had to arise in Haiti. The first relates to identity. The second pertains to the views people have regarding the body and death.

First, with regard to identity, at the time of death an individual can pretend to be his own father, his grandfather, or his cousin . . . because there is a real problem in Haiti with regard to personal records. Many people are born, live, and die without ever having obtained legal existence. They thus disappear without having ever existed (in the eyes of the national registry). Therefore, it is quite possible to change lives by affirming that so-and-so has died, then openly taking his place within the rest of the family, which accepts this impersonation with kindness, or at least with neutrality (in the same way as in the film *Le Retour de Martin Guerre,* or as with Jeanne des Armoises, who, having assumed the identity of Joan of Arc after the latter's execution by burning in 1431, succeeded in being acknowledged by Joan of Arc's brothers). This adoption of individuals can happen slowly and in stages, like an agreement that enables one to solve a problem arising within a clan, such as a lack of manpower, a lack of financial means, a "shameful" illness, etc. But this case remains rare. Normally, the individual considered to be a zombie wanders throughout the land, is characterized by abnormal social behavior, and ends up at the crossroads or along the roadway without any possessions. It is his recognition by a third party that will give him the name of zombie (and no longer only a vagabond) and will turn him into a being that is spiritually separate. But we must understand that a complete investigation risks showing that the zombie is never dead, no more so than if he were drugged, and that he may be no more than someone who took advantage of a death to occupy a place left vacant because it was beneficial to him or to the community, and that he "whitens" or "supports" this identity shift under the term and the concept of zombification. This position is facilitated by the fantasy that is present in a widespread and diffuse manner within Haiti that zombies move among the living.

Next, a word about the body. From the beginning of Haitian history, as a result of the slave trade and slavery, the body of men is a stolen body. It is a body uprooted from the African soil and forcibly brought to the island of Saint-Domingue from 1517 under the impetus of Charles V. The individual begins by carrying out a certain number of activities to recover his body, such as the struggle led by slaves to escape this servile condition. We must go beyond the surface level of acts of war and become interested in the efforts made by men to reclaim themselves. It is there where one touches the sacred and where Haitian Vodou intercedes. This religious system is founded on the fact that, in death, man rejoins Africa (called *Afrique-Guinée*), and thus the spirits and gods of origin. A symbolic chain has been broken by slavery, a chain that links the individual, the family, the dead, the ancestors, and gods. This is why the cult of the dead (*guédé*) is one of the most important within Haitian Vodou, to which slaves were tied very early from their first enrollment in the Dominican system. It is there to fill an absence and to reestablish the individual's own roots. This preeminence still persists. The individual needs to consolidate the spiritual forces that enable his body to be a true human body. Because a body that does not have a protective force available is only a mound of flesh with which one can do anything (turn it into an animal, for example) and constitutes an extremely dangerous situation. Starting from the African system of anthropology of the body, there is an upping of the ante, an overinvestment of the very vision of the spiritual forces that protect the body, because of this forced removal, this violent separation from the homeland.[7]

But of what is this body made? First, it is a pile of flesh around which two spiritual elements are structured. The first (*petit bon ange* or *ti-bon-anj*) corresponds to the intrinsic part of the individual that is in contact with spirits (*loas*), memory, consciousness, and authority. It travels during the night in the form of dreams, meets spirits, and obtains a certain quantity of knowledge about itself and its family, but also about talents (for healing, for example). The *petit bon ange* can leave the body of the individual at the moment of possession by the *loa*. It detaches itself from the earthly body in order to give the *loa* room to move in and take possession of the subject. The second (*gros bon ange* or *gwo-bon-anj*) corresponds to intelligence and will (the motor principle). Once a person has been initiated into Vodou, a part of the *loa* (to which he or she has been consecrated) stays permanently within the individual. But certain Vodou practitioners can go even farther and obtain more divinities. For example, they can put all or part of their *petit bon ange* (or their *gros bon ange*) in a bottle placed under the protection of a peristyle (Haitian Vodou temple) so that no one with evil intentions will capture it (that is to say, steal it during death or before, during the process of zombification). For the initiate, there is thus a great risk of theft of this spiritual element, or of insertion of an element in him that would be a source of unrest within his own body and that would disrupt his spirit. Hence, the devout person spends his time preventing others from assuming his identity, which explains the countless practical rituals that give their tempo to Haitian daily life in the form of offensive and defensive magic. The individual is not, in fact, obsessed with death, but with the struggle against his own premature death, which could occur at any instant.

For historical and contextual reasons, the Haitian system is a system of economic and social violence. With a population of over 10 million people, life expectancy is only 61 years for both men and women. The fertility rate is 3.81 children per female, but the infant mortality rate is extremely high, with nearly 60 deaths per one thousand births (compared to 3.37 in France). Overall, 60 percent of the population is less than 25 years of age. It must be said that as soon as one walks in the streets, whether in the capital or in the scrubland, they are full of schoolchildren in uniform. On the other hand, as soon as a Haitian gets white hair, they saddle him with jeers like "gramps," "the old one," and "hippie."

In this context in which death is so frequent, everyone can see or imagine individuals everywhere who are capable of killing or of stealing a spirit. At certain key moments, crises can arise and make one believe that there are numerous and widespread secret societies, that systematized pillaging of cemeteries occurs, or even that there is a plethora of zombies. The earthquake of January 12, 2010 (which caused more than 230,000 deaths), like all disasters or times of crisis, was a time of real inflation in zombification cases: many zombies were reported in the refugee camps. Sociologists and religion scholars were expecting this; in Haiti, the supernatural world is continually present. To borrow Alice Corbet's expression, "invisible beings [are] omnipresent"[8] (speaking of those who disappeared during the quake). In fact, there were no individual funerals for these victims, who were usually buried hastily in common graves. Furthermore, not all bodies were found, and many remained under the rubble. They were thereafter covered over by new construction, outside of all sepulchral context, and thus without any accompanying ritual.

In general, the Haitian population—all generations combined—has a complete belief in zombies, and it is difficult to convince anyone that this phenomenon does not exist. And when one asks Laënnec Hurbon the question to find out whether he believes in zombies, he answers without answering: "I believe that people, because they are schizophrenic, can return at a certain time to the structure of the mythology of zombification, and that they declare themselves 'zombies.' I believe that that is what happens most often." It is true that *bokors* use toxic substances to conduct a certain number of both offensive and counteroffensive magical activities, because clients come to ask them to resolve such and such a problem with such and such a person (a resolution that is as symbolic and it is real, effective, and tangible). With zombies, there is a mixture of things relating not only to everyday toxicity (plants, animals, etc.), but also to other magical-religious elements (a twin system of real and fantasy). At all crossroads, in every cemetery, at the foot of all imposing trees, one sees *roga*—that is, magical objects targeting a very specific individual. And when this individual passes in front or nearby, he understands immediately that this spell is directed at him. Then, he falls ill (sympathetically—that is, without even having either touched or drunk anything). In turn, he must go to consult a *houngan* (Vodou priest practicing good magic) in order to find the cure for this spell and to undo it by the use of counter-magic. There thus exists a spectrum of practices that range from totally benign gestures to the extreme case or limit that zombification embodies. This blueprint is already present within society, and society chooses whether or not to exploit it.

It is when the masses correctly identify a zombie that one notices this real familiarity with death within the Haitian people. People are almost too comfortable with this phenomenon, and evolve naturally with it. On the other hand, few dare to touch it (at the risk of being contaminated in some way), for this would almost be touching death. As soon as he is identified as a zombie, the individual is led to the church so that a priest can "place a cord" around him—in other words, allow him to return to daily life. A sort of new baptism following a rebirth, since the individual has known death and has returned from it, it consists of a sprinkling of holy water. Catholic baptism is indeed integrated into the Vodou system as an additional force required for the *loa* to function correctly. Since the individual is not possessed but, on the contrary, deprived of his soul, this is definitely not an exorcism, but rather a purifying bath. Through these ceremonies, there is an attempt to make the stolen *petit bon ange* (*ti-bon-anj*) return. It comes back gradually, in stages. We see here a phenomenon relating to a twin system of real and fantasy that is interconnected within the Haitian anthropological view.

In Vodou temples, collected in a room away from the pathway, one frequently sees fetishes or numerous bottles bordering an altar. They are filled with the souls of the living or of the dead, and they serve as protection (in theory, nothing can happen—neither capture, nor zombification—to the individual who has put his soul in contact with *loas*). Tradition says that when one tries to lift these bottles (these are ordinary old 50 to 100 cl. wine or rum bottles), any movement is impossible. *Houngans* and Vodou practitioners say that they are so "filled with souls" that they cannot even be tipped or removed them from the ground. Nobody can move them. In any case, no one except for priests has the right to touch them. That's the Gospel truth.

Nowadays, Haitians have such fear of being zombified that they take off and convert to Protestantism (mainly to the new Pentecostal and Baptist movements reserved for the working classes; more rarely Methodist, but also Mormon and Jehovah's Witnesses). They thus believe themselves to be protected, impregnable, and beyond all magic. In fact, and without expecting it, Protestants are revitalizing the entire Vodou imagination, because Haitians, knowing that the social situation has completely degenerated (especially since the earthquake of 2010), now think that any normal person is vulnerable. It is for this reason that Vodou is necessarily forsaken and demonized at the time of conversion. This moment of demonization of Vodou is yet another way of keeping it alive, since it grants it both a real existence and real power. In sermons, it is necessary always to talk about Vodou, to declare that it is evil, dangerous, a source of conflict and death, and above all, the cause of all misfortunes on the island (*sic!*). Consequently, many Haitians spend their time frequenting all types of churches; they need that in order to feel protected. But are they really? That is the question. In any case, they are afraid of neither *houngans* nor *bokors.*

When one asks where the zombies are during the day and whether they work on the plantations, Haitians answer in the most serious way in the world: "They are there, but you can't see them because they disappear from the view of others." Conversely, in the evening, at nightfall, zombies are gathered there. They eat off banana leaves (they do not eat like humans, but like slaves, for they are on the brink of death), and the following morning, everything starts all over again. This way of seeing and then no longer seeing the zombie shows that one is in a shared fantasy, with one part of the imagination that is extremely important to the meaning of zombification.

Land or marital disputes, professional jealousies, and lawsuits are potential sources for zombie creation. Parents can even zombify their children . . . unless it is about nothing more than a simple swindle? Thus, in Terrier-Rouge (on the northeast side of the island), a false zombification recently occurred (2010)—a very successful staging by a *houngan* seeking to prove that he had extraordinary abilities, particularly the power "to raise the dead." He thus did so with his own son, who played the role to near-perfection.

CHAPTER 4

AN OVERVIEW OF HAITIAN VODOU

Since the 1920s, both local and foreign university studies have made it possible to understand the organization and the mysticism of Haitian Vodou in a very specific way.[1] These animistic beliefs are founded on the transmission of *Yoruba* magical-religious content from West Africa by means of the slave trade, including and especially through the intermediary of music.[2] First and foremost, the word *Vodou* means "spirit" or "divinity":

> In the Fon language spoken in Benin, *vodun* means invisible, frightful and mysterious power having the ability to intervene at any moment within the society of humans. The deportation of millions of slaves to the New World brought about the re-formation of African beliefs and practices in the Americas in diverse forms and terms: Candomblé in Brazil, Santería in Cuba, Obeah in Jamaica, Shango cult in Trinity, or Vodou in Haiti. . . . Facing a pro-slavery system that claims to remove them completely from their humanity, little by little, Blacks deported from Africa devise their own religion through the rites of Vodou. This is a radical fantasy at the same time as it is a real community link that will constitute the clandestine cornerstone of their various struggles for freedom.[3]

Followers of Vodou (*hounsi*) are grouped within a *société* whose seat is located in a *hounfor* in which rituals guided by priests and priestesses called *houngan* and *mambo*, respectively, are performed.

Baptism, which French colonists imposed on their slaves and which introduced them to their new condition of servitude, was very quickly interpreted as a new door of entry to Vodou rituals. At the same time, this baptism, and also mandatory Catholic education, have been at the origins of this very particular syncretism between Christianity and the traditional religions of Black Africa. In the end, the *loas*, these tribal divinities, have more or less been likened to Catholic saints. The integration has been so strong that Marian statues, Black Virgins, candles, and sacred relics have also been incorporated into rituals.[4]

Loas are very active in religious life and often possess followers through trance episodes:

> The explanation given by Vodou sect members regarding the mystical trance is very simple. A *loa* stays inside the head of an individual after having chased from it the *gwo-bon anj*, one of the two souls that each individual carries within him- or herself. It is the abrupt departure of the soul that causes the shudders and spasms characteristic of the beginning of a trance. Once the *bon anj* has left, the possessed person experiences the feeling of complete emptiness, as if he were losing consciousness. His head turns and the hollows of his knees tremble. He then becomes not only the receptacle of God, but also his instrument. It is the personality of God and no longer his own that he expresses in his words. . . . The relationship that exists between the *loa* and the man of whom it takes hold is equivalent to the one that connects the horseman to his mount.[5]

Indeed, they say that the *loa* "rides his servant," that takes the form of the spirit that dominates him. Thus, during his convulsions on the ground, a *hounsi* ridden by Damballa will stick his tongue out of his mouth like a snake. Rituals are performed to pay homage to *loas* (literally while "feeding" them—*manjé-loa*) with the stated goal of bringing luck to oneself.

Secret societies are characterized by the carrying out under the cloak of the Vodou religion of activities normally deemed malevolent (which is the source, for some people, of the poor reputation given to this religion). These societies are called Bizango, Cochon gris, etc. They say that they practice human and cannibalistic sacrifices (which is, in all likelihood, exaggerated), particularly at the time of possession by protective totemic animals (*baka*). The latter are types of evil spirits that frequently assume animal forms such as a werewolf, leopard-man, snake-man, elephant-man, owl-man, crocodile-man, and lion-man. We see that the vast majority of these animal species are not prevalent within Haiti and that they originate from an African source (a subconscious background). Some even take the form of invisible birds detectable at night only by their bright trail, if not the odor of sulfur from their wake. Throughout the Haitian dictatorship, the Duvaliers—father and son—(1957–1986) maintained suspicion regarding the true nature of their militia, the Tontons Macoutes, which the majority of Haitians considered to be members of these secret societies gifted with particularly dangerous magical powers.

Bokors, those who serve the *loas* "with their two hands," are *houngans* who have decided to do both good and evil magic (especially participating in zombification rituals or even in the consecration of *ouangas*—or *wangas*—these dangerous talismans—magical packets—lodging *baka*). The *angajan* is the magical-religious pact signed between a believer and a *loa* that has harmful intentions for someone.

In the Vodou religion, human beings are made up of five basic elements: body (the flesh that becomes the corpse after death), *n'âme* (the spirit that animates the flesh and which, also mortal, becomes an energy transmitted to the earth at the time of death), *z'étoile* (the star of destiny that lives in paradise at a distance away from the body), and *gwo-bon-anj* and *ti-bon-anj* (the two parts of the soul). Within the magical-religious concept of Haitian Vodou, death is not the end of life, but the change from one state to another. If the body, in fact, decomposes, if the *n'âme* disappears into the depths of the ground, the *gwo-bon-anj* meets the sun and *Ginen* (the cosmic community of ancestral spirits) to become a *loa*, while the *ti-bon-anj* is confined to the kingdom of the dead.

The *ti-bon-anj* does not indeed immediately leave the corpse at the moment of death, but hovers around it for nine days that are concluded with a ceremony called "On the ninth evening." This ceremony ends by interring the *ti-bon-anj* within the tomb, the true gateway to the sojourn of the dead. If this ritual is not practiced, there is a risk that the *ti-bon-anj* will wander on earth and will cause misfortunes to the friends of the departed. Through a magical process, the *houngan* can thus force the *ti-bon-anj* to remain a year and a day within the murky waters of a lake before the family ritually calls it back. Transformed into a spirit, it is placed in a *govi* (a jar covered in necklaces) that will be either specially dedicated to the religion (thus fed and worshiped in the same way as any *loa*), or broken and its fragments distributed over several crossroads (to free the spirit and to allow it to enter the land of the dead).

Another magical process performed by the *houngan*, the *dessounin* (or *desounen*) enables the *gwo-bon-anj* to separate from the dead body. The nostrils and the ears of the deceased are closed with cotton, while the knees and big toes are tied together, the mouth is closed, and the pockets of his or her clothing are turned inside out. Next, the *houngan* throws local rum (*clairin*) both to the four compass points and on the body in order to purify it, shakes his *asson*[6] on the corpse, and lights candles. The *asson* is a rattle belonging to the *houngan* or the *mambo* consisting of a calabash covered with a net in the mesh of which grains of porcelain or garter snake vertebra are inserted (a royal attribute and symbol of power). Then the name of the deceased is whispered into the *houngan*'s ears while his assistants perform animal sacrifices and trace the *vévés* consecrated to the dead (those of Baron Samedi or Dame Brigitte, for example). Often, the *houngan* is possessed by the spirit of the dead, and this trance is the opportunity to foresee the future of the deceased's close family. Until this ritual (*desounen*) is completed, the deceased is still considered to be living.

Of course, there are ways to invert these ceremonies into something evil. To perform a *prise du mort*, a *bokor* goes into a cemetery, calls upon Baron Samedi to obtain the authorization to bring a soul out from a grave, then throws rum on a funerary stone while placing a few coins on it, and finally strikes the headstone with a calabash. In similar fashion, the *bokor* can also steal the *ti-bon-anj* during this fateful period of the nine days following death. In the event of capture (in a bottle), this spirit becomes what the Haitians call a *zombi astral*. Contrary to the traditional zombie, there is no tangible dimension (it is a bodiless spirit from which the *bokor* can command numerous and varied actions and which will never find rest).

How can someone actually prevent a *bokor*'s potential harmful doings? How can one ensure that the dead body will not be desecrated and that the souls will not be carried away? Ideally, the family must not leave the cemetery until the deceased is completely buried inside his sepulcher, out of fear of bodysnatching (and thus out of fear of possible zombification). In morgues, if there is doubt about the "real and consistent" nature of death, Laënnec Hurbon tells me that some people manage to "kill the individual a second time"[7] (the body is not beheaded, for the deceased must be presentable to the family or to the public during viewing in the church; therefore all visible mutilation is avoided, so poison or a stab right in the heart is used instead). One can also resort to magical practices: in scattering eyeless needles and balls of wool within the grave, for example, or even several thousand sesame seeds, it is believed that the spirit of the dead will be so busy with these impossible tasks that it will not hear the voice of the *bokor* instructing it to exit the grave. Still others position a knife in the hand of the corpse so that he might plant it in the heart of the *bokor* or those of his assistants at the moment of exhumation. Noticing that a dead body's nails have been cut or hair pulled out is, on the other hand, an undeniable sign that a *bokor* is in the process of casting a spell on this deceased person.

CHAPTER 5

FIRST HAITIAN CEMETERY

With Laënnec Hurbon on board, our car sinks into the sugar cane plantations and rolls past shuttered factories. After an hour, we reach the cemetery near the Digneron colonial sugar plantation. Half-starved goats are wandering amid the gravesites. Wild grasses are growing on the graves, and the noise of trucks loaded with sugar cane is deafening.

The place is telling of Haitians' own thoughts on the fate of the deceased: the dead must be shut up and cemented tightly (even if no encompassing wall delimits the cemetery, strictly speaking). Many vaults are thus sealed off with iron doors locked by huge padlocks because the theft of caskets (in order to reuse them), possessions of the deceased, and body parts is frequent. Primarily it is skulls that are stolen, because many magical practices are focused on this specific anatomical part, which has great symbolic importance. Many rituals take place in the cemeteries because they are under the authority of the *loa* Baron Samedi, leader of death and of both offensive and defensive magical practices.

On the pathways or between the gravestones, several opened caskets are visible, on which chickens climb in search of food. A child's casket, completely white, is overturned and empty. Corpses have been stolen, either within a magical context, or as a result of simple vandalism (degradation of worship). More and more, one is under the impression that there is a decrease in respect in Haiti with regard to the dead. When everything becomes an occasion for depredation, it suggests that the culture is experiencing a crisis that touches the very foundations of society: the taboo associated with the dead. It is within this ferment that the fantasy of zombification largely germinates. Some vaults are wide open (animals seek refuge there to flee the heat). While casting a glance at one of them, I see the scattered bones of a child, some scraps of clothing, bottles of alcohol, and several offerings made to the *guédés* or to Baron Samedi (calabashes, coconuts bound together, and candles).

At the exit of the cemetery, in the yard of a private home, a strange object is hung from a tree. It is a small wicker chair, about thirty centimeters high, to which a bright red doll and a few food offerings are tied. The entire thing, which is about three meters (ten feet) high, has its back to the house. It is the result of a very practical Vodou ritual designed to destroy those who gaze too closely at a family or an individual. At the end of a brief ceremony, we "put the other back in his place" by issuing the following order to him: "Sit down there. Don't move any more. You are watching me too much." This is Vodou pragmatism. Instead of killing him, you symbolically chain him as if you had said to him, "Remain calm, my dear friend. . . ." The target can be represented by a doll (as in the present instance), a stone, a photograph, a lock of hair, etc.

CHAPTER 6

MAX BEAUVOIR

On the roadside of the national highway that runs to the south toward Jacmel, a sign that reads, "Peristyle Mariani" sits on top of a wrought-iron porch. Nestled in an immense park, Max Beauvoir's house adjoins his Vodou sanctuary. Designed by him, this house is magical, "organic," and curvy. Books are spread out on all of the walls alongside sculptures polished by time, old furniture, and a few good-luck charms. Night falls when our conversation begins. Seated at a table outside under a mango tree, very quickly overwhelmed by mosquitoes and the evening drizzle, we seek refuge in his office near a fan of painted metal sheeting.

Due to his stature, authority, warm voice, beautiful, muscular hands, his wrinkles and white hair, and his publications, Max Beauvoir commands respect. All of this together means that he lives on these premises with an incredible intensity. He is a *houngan*, but due to his training, he has a very biological (and, as it happens, very toxicological) view of the phenomenon of zombies. For several years, he has been an *ati*—in other words, the supreme ruler of Haitian Vodou, thus in charge of this religious and cultural tradition of the Haitian people. As a guardian of this culture, he is forced always to have the practice of Vodou in hand, while also maintaining a naturalistic view of it, through plants, nature, people, and their interconnections. "By combining the two," affirms Max Beauvoir, "it may be possible to understand first what man is, then life, and how this life is made (with this dual element of the physical and the spiritual)." There are so many things that are not taught in schools, but that, for him, give life its full meaning.

Before becoming a *houngan*, Max Beauvoir was trained as a biochemist. He completed his studies in New York (City College), in Paris (Sorbonne), and in Reims (School of Science), and upon returning to the United States, at Cornell University, with a thesis in chemistry. Back in Haiti, he continued his doctoral work by researching hydrocortisone within plants, which led him to file a patent in this area. Strictly limited to the United States, this patent brings him nothing at all! His daughter, Rachel, pursued the same path in anthropology and became a *mambo*. It was not Max who initiated her, but her spiritual father, André Basquiat.

Max Beauvoir was "revealed" to the Western world in 1985 in a publication authored by Canadian ethnobotanist Wade Davis. In 1981, Nathan Kline, whom Beauvoir had known at Cornell University (New York Hospital), calls Max to ask him a favor: he wants to know even more about zombies. Max then invites a young scientist (Wade Davis) to come spend some time with him to begin research on this phenomenon. Here is how Davis sums up his Haitian experience: "My mission, such as was briefly described by Kline, was to go to Haiti to find Vodou sorcerers responsible [for zombification] and to obtain poison and antidote samples from them while observing their preparation and, if possible, document their use. . . ."[1] This is what he did for just a few weeks during the summer of 1982. He paid a lot of money for several samples, justifying his purchases at times as purely for scientific research, and at other times as due to his desire to "get rid of an enemy."

This exchange with the North American professor enabled Max Beauvoir to expand his own view on zombies, which was very Haitian at first. With this dual ethnological/scientific perspective (practical and logical), he was able to carry out research that was much more original. Without taking all of the precautions of modern scientists, Haitian *bokors*, even if they were unaware of it, were also involved in chemistry. For example, they were making their toxic powders on a portable kitchen stove while protecting themselves only with a handkerchief over the nose, while the best American laboratories risk handling such dangerous molecules only under fume hoods, in safety suits, etc.

For several weeks, Wade Davis, accompanied by Max Beauvoir and his daughter, explored the toxic products present on the island and in the neighboring waters. He focused his interest on a fish called *fufu* in Haitian (the equivalent of *fugu* in Japan), and tetraodon by scientists. The poison developed from this animal is thus called tetrodotoxin. It is nothing more than a blowfish that, when frightened, has the ability to swell itself up quickly with water and become enormous, while raising the spines on its sides. Within this fish, at the level of its skin, is a particularly toxic substance that Japanese chefs know well, some of them having blacked out while they were preparing this dish (when it hasn't been a customer who became ill from ingesting it . . .). It has become necessary for chefs to obtain special certification in order to prepare and sell this fish in a restaurant. Clinical symptoms are nearly identical whether one swallows the organs of this fish or the powder extracted from them is absorbed through the victim's skin. According to what Wade Davis and Max Beauvoir learned from their anthropological and toxicological investigation, but also from Japanese evidence collected by a Dr. Kao, a set of symptoms slowing down vital functions temporarily settles into the person's system, leading as far as catalepsy (syncope)—in other words, up to a state of apparent death. In the absence of appropriate treatment, the victim ultimately dies.

Here in Haiti, Wade Davis and Max Beauvoir conducted another experiment. For the first time, they had evidence that zombies were not the fruit of fantasies or a simple literary creation, but that they truly existed. Previously, no one had scientifically described either the presence or the reality of zombies. There had always been a number of go-betweens insisting that they'd known someone who had seen a zombie, etc. At the conclusion of their investigation, Davis and Beauvoir succeeded in having the existence of such individuals, transformed by drugs, recognized officially and by the international scientific community. At the center of their evidence is a man named Clairvius Narcisse, who was found in a market in Artibonite (in the northern part of the island) several years after his "death." Scientifically speaking, this man, whom Davis and Beauvoir studied from every angle (as they did his family), can be considered zombie #1. His complete history has been taken, as have medical observations, whether concerning his death certificate, his funeral, his public inhumation (which was attested by many credible witnesses), his exhumation, his transit through hospitals, etc. The real toxicological research began when they sought to find out how Clairvius Narcisse became this zombie.

At the beginning of this investigation, it seemed logical to me to believe that when one is a *houngan* (or a *bokor*, that is, a priest favoring black magic), zombies are almost part of daily life, and something to which one is accustomed. I naively imagined that when this sort of Vodou priest completes his professional apprenticeship, he is taught the current and traditional methods of zombification. In short, one course is like any other. I certainly did not think that this was lawful, nor even good, but I imagined that this existed, at least within the apprenticeship. This view—Western?—is completely erroneous to Max Beauvoir, for whom there is no learning to make zombies, either at the time of initiation or indeed at any moment of the initiate life. The person who is zombified is someone who has received a punishment for bad behavior (asocial or antisocial behavior). A judgment is brought down by a group of elders who possess genuine importance within the Haitian community.

In the case of Clairvius Narcisse, such a judgment was pronounced after the death of his father, who had left him a plot of land that Clairvius, the eldest of the family, wanted to sell in order to collect the money and leave for the United States (Miami, like many Haitians do). At the time, everyone had tried to discourage him, because this small plot served to provide for his entire family. But he persisted, and he asked for the help of law enforcement in taking possession of the land for the purpose of selling it as planned. It was then that he was judged by what they call "the Society" (the "Secret Society" of anthropologists or, as Max Beauvoir prefers to call it, "The Sacred Society") in order to dissuade him. But as Clairvius still insisted, this group had no other choice but to turn him into a zombie. And he remained a zombie for several years until Wade Davis and Max Beauvoir came to "disturb" him and to make him emerge from this condition little by little, even to the point of giving him back his full status among the living. Clairvius Narcisse even brought them to visit his vault—an open tomb—in Estère cemetery (near Artibonite). He told them how a nail from the casket had partly torn his cheek (the skin of which still shows the scar). There were so many supporting arguments—in addition to the testimonies of his loved ones who physically recognized him—that it was, in fact, definitely him. Dr. Leslie Desmangles had indeed raised the possibility of identity theft, because the body of Clairvius Narcisse would have been refrigerated for approximately twenty hours before his burial, which would have made his survival unlikely, including after a massive dose of poisons.

Wade Davis was the advocate for a single poison used for zombification (he had even already found the name of it: "poison zombie" or "zombinol"). But Max Beauvoir, who, by nature, knows the Haitian soul better, attempted to explain to him that he was heading down the wrong path and that the problem was much more complex. Davis, it seems to him, failed to realize that to understand zombies, one has to include the spiritual part of man, or at least the way in which Haitians view and think of man. Of course, man has a body. But he also has a soul. If saying this is easy, then living it each day as a "spirit with a body" proves to be quite different. It is to be largely spirit, of the same nature as God, and the body, in what is us, is nothing more than "the seeds of an apple," to borrow Max Beauvoir's expression. Thus, man (the apple) is much more than what one thinks he is, and he does not reduce himself to this biased view that we usually have of him.

At the conclusion of his fieldwork, and of testing conducted in the United States on samples collected from *bokors* and patients *in situ*, Davis could nonetheless identify roughly five different methods permitting the more or less successful zombification of an individual, even if, as Max Beauvoir clarifies, drugs do not do everything. For him, psychology, education, and societal pressure participate in nearly equal proportions in the creation of a zombie. These five substances gathered throughout Haitian territory always contain common points in their compositions, starting with the *fufu* fish.

The concept of zombies is thus at the convergence of toxicology, medicine, magic, and religion. A zombie is a follower of Vodou who, on account of bad behavior, has been judged and then convicted by the secret societies. Within other chrono-cultural contexts, "we would use either a gun or a rope to solve the problem," says Max Beauvoir with a big, disarming smile. But in this case, a solution worse than death is chosen: zombification. In other words, the destruction of an active life is replaced by the survival of an individual deprived of all decision-making power (a "vegetable"). It is a solution against those who act badly. One "moves the *petit-bon-ange*," this spiritual part of the human being that makes the individual intelligent and free to make his or her own choices. As soon as it is moved, the person will still exist, but will no longer desire to do evil. From then on, he or she can be released or entrusted to others. The person will no longer cause any problems to society. He will definitely not be able to make a living, but if his family recognizes him, it is free to take him back into its custody until his death. Clairvius Narcisse took full advantage of his "new life," supported by the sisters of Passe-Reine (in the highlands of Artibonite), and having benefited from numerous American visas granted him in order to make sightseeing tours and university visits . . . but also to meet his second wife (eighteen years of age when he was already over fifty!), and even to have new children and to end up dying a quiet death! This is proof that zombies can have a second life, and even a full one.

The evangelists made a lot of hay of these beliefs in zombies, and were even pleased to say that the 2010 earthquake was a divine punishment in response to Vodou practitioners who "serve Satan and play with death." They began to create false zombies themselves in the north of Haiti, with stereotypical, even cartoonish, stories, with the goal of making fun of Vodou practitioners and extending their own sphere of evangelism.

I speak to Max Beauvoir of Vodou followers who attempt to shield themselves from zombification by having a part of themselves enclosed in bottles safeguarded within a peristyle. It does not seem possible to him to rob people of their "soul," even in the form of a *ti-bon-anj* in a flask or a bottle. "How would a man have the power to undo what God has done? As in all religions, that does not work within Vodou," he says wisely. This does not prevent man from taking himself for a demiurge from time to time, but Max Beauvoir does not tell everything, and does not publicly admit to believing in the effectiveness of these ceremonies and places of protection for souls in danger. "It is literature that is a bit exaggerated . . . ," is all he will say. But does he believe what he says?

CHAPTER 7

TETRODOTOXIN

The weather is bad in Port-au-Prince. A tropical shower is pouring down on the city and its surrounding areas. The sky over the Caribbean Sea is totally overcast, and not a single boat is leaving port. Not even the massive ocean liners. It is the ideal moment to shut oneself away in the library in what remains of the School of Medicine. While the streets sink into a deep darkness, a long bibliographic search on outdated computers in the patched-up stacks enlightens me little by little on this strange substance called tetrodotoxin (TTX).

This molecule, whose exact chemical formula is $C_{11}H_{17}N_3O_8$, is an extremely toxic product found in several rare aquatic animals from tropical regions,[1] such as blowfish (*Lagocephalus scleratus*/*Tetraodon stellatus*/*Diodon hystrix*/*Spheroides testudineus*, etc.; the liver, skin, eyes and gonads of these fish are particularly rich in poison, while the muscles, except when contaminated by the previously named anatomic zones, are harmless)[2], octopuses (*Hapalochlaena lunulata*, *H. maculosa*),[3] gastropods, crabs,[4] amphibians (poison dart frog, salamander),[5] etc.

It would seem that it is not the blowfish that synthesizes this toxin (to which it is indeed resistant), but the bacteria (*Pseudomonas*) found in red algae (*Rhodophyta*).[6] While eating, the fish accumulates this toxin and stores it in its organs.[7]

Intoxication by tetrodotoxin usually shows a progression of rather stereotypical clinical indicators.[8] Level 1: Pins and needles (paresthesia) around the mouth, with gastrointestinal problems, including stomach pain, nausea, vomiting, heartburn, diarrhea, etc. Level 2: Pins and needles (paresthesia) through the torso and the extremities, with appearance of paralysis and difficulty with coordination of movement. Level 3: Diffused paralysis, arterial hypotension, and aphasia. Level 4: Loss of consciousness, paralysis of respiratory muscles, severe arterial hypotension, and disturbance of cardiac rhythm. Simultaneously, hypothermia as well as a significant slowing of heartbeats can occur, in such a way that the clinical situation resembles that of a state of apparent death.[9] With the improvement of diagnostic criteria and resuscitation techniques, when poisoning is detected, mortality, which exceeded eighty percent at the beginning of the 20th century, is today around thirty percent.[10] There are still, however, around fifty deaths in Japan each year, despite the preparation of *fugu* by master chefs required to obtain specific certification prior to offering this dish in their restaurants.[11] The consumption of this fish (*fufu* or *fugu*) is so dangerous that the emperor of Japan and samurai, they say, were forbidden to taste it (this ban still exists for the Japanese sovereign). No effective treatment has thus far been identified, although Datura (*Datura stramonium*) and strychnine were suggested at one time.[12]

For some individuals, in a sort of game with death, the last word in Japanese gastronomy means leaving a small piece of liver in contact with the meat of the *fugu* in order for the customer to feel a bit of tingling on the lips (corresponding to level 1 of tetrodotoxin poisoning).

In 1975, a famous Japanese actor of *nô* theatre (Bando Mitsugoro VIII) died after having eaten four servings of *fugu kimo* (blowfish liver) in a Kyoto restaurant. Out of bravado, this living national treasure had claimed that he was capable of surviving the ingestion of this dish whose sale is forbidden. After having finished his plate and those of three of his guests, he died in his hotel room after seven hours of agony marked by convulsions and paralysis.

Since then, numerous cases of tetrodotoxin poisoning have been described in the scientific literature: twenty-seven poisonings (two fatal) in Brazil between 1984 and 2009,[13] seven poisonings in Hong Kong (one fatal) in 1995,[14] one non-fatal poisoning in Taiwan in 1995,[15] three non-fatal poisonings in California in 1996,[16] one non-fatal poisoning in Malaysia in 1997,[17] one non-fatal poisoning in Australia in 1998,[18] fifty-three poisonings (six fatal) in Bangladesh between 2001 and 2006[19] with thirty-seven poisonings (eight fatal) in 2002,[20] nine deaths in Cambodia in the Sihanoukville region between 2003 and 2007,[21] six poisonings (two fatal) in Taiwan in 2005,[22] three non-fatal poisonings in Malaysia in 2006,[23] two poisonings in Japan in 2008 in the province of Nagasaki,[24] sixty-three poisonings (fourteen fatal) in Bangladesh in 2008,[25] etc.

Until the 1980s, neither ethnologists nor the local Haitian population specifically connected the tradition of zombies to simple magical practices or to the use of a still-unknown substance. Everything changed in 1983 with the publication of a sensational article signed by Canadian ethnobotanist Wade David,[26] followed by the launch of a book aimed at the general public,[27] then by the defense of his thesis.[28] The hypothesis he defends is that of criminal poisoning of human subjects via decoctions containing tetrodotoxin at a sub-lethal dosage. In other words, the dosage is enough to send the victim into a state of apparent death, justifying a funeral followed by inhumation, before the body is recovered *a posteriori*, resuscitated, and then socially considered to be a zombie.

Some colleagues question the validity of this hypothesis.[29] They maintain that the concentration of tetrodotoxin is too variable from one sample to another,[30] and that it almost never produces the expected yields.[31] In other words, the experiment is not reproducible. If Davis did not test the effectiveness of such substances on a healthy man, he did, on the other hand, induce a deep sleep in Dr. Léon Roisin's lab rats (New York State Psychiatric Institute) by injecting them in the peritoneum with the product obtained from a Haitian *bokor*. All things being equal, several environmental factors can explain the significant variation in concentration (and thus the effectiveness or the delay of action) of *poudre à zombi* collected by Wade Davis or analyzed by the cohort of ethnobiologists who followed him: first, seasonality in the production and storage of tetrodotoxin by the blowfish; then, the gradual transformation (by humidity, by variation of pH) of the powder between its synthesis and its use. Finally, as Wade Davis quite rightly mentions, any psychoactive drug has a completely unpredictable potential within it. Pharmacologically, it induces a certain state, a simple raw material that will be transformed, in particular, by forces and the cultural or psychological expectations of the subject and of the society that surrounds him or her.

It is what the experts call "set and setting" within any drug-taking experiment. "Set" corresponds to the expectations of what the medicine is going to do to the individual; "Setting" relates to the environment—both physical and, in this case, social—in which the substance is consumed.[32]

Except that tetrodotoxin is not a psychoactive drug because it seldom crosses the blood-brain barrier (the separation between the vascular system and the central nervous system), and the possible neuro-psychological effects that it can have are only peripheral (acting on the nervous system separate from the brain and spinal cord) or linked to distress of the brain tissue caused by overly low vascularization or oxygenation of the blood.[33]

Max Beauvoir recalls that he had been contacted by NASA in 1983 to put astronauts in a state of catalepsy during tentative flights to Mars. Its engineers had, indeed, thought of being able to "zombify" these astronauts during their long navigation by using the products described by Davis and Beauvoir in Haiti. This idea was not pursued. Other scientists who were more realistic thought of introducing tetrodotoxin into molecular cocktails for extended local anesthetics[34] or analgesics.[35]

CHAPTER 8

MY FIRST ZOMBIE

Jacques Ravix is my first patient in Haiti, but because he is a gynecologist, he is also my colleague. In 1994, he went "to the other side," and since his accident, he has retained a few neurological effects, including significant dysarthria and difficulty walking.

As he says, he has lived "some very peculiar moments."[1] In 1974, at 33 years of age and married, with three children, he had just returned from France (the Schools of Medicine in Montpellier and Besançon, where he defended his thesis).[2] He practiced medicine as a generalist and as a gynecologist in a maternity ward in Port-au-Prince. Then he strung together other jobs at the tax office and even at the Department of Justice (they were lacking middle managers at the time). In 1994, at age 53, he ran into problems with his spouse that were so substantial that they ended up separating. The mother of this woman sought retaliation against Jacques Ravix, and had him poisoned by tetrodotoxin.

At the scientific and professional levels, Jacques knew this poison well. He had already seen several of his patients die within only a few hours following an acute poisoning. But a chronic, slow, insidious dosage is also possible until it reaches the intended effect: to render a person neither living nor dead. The individual survives, but does not even know what he is doing. He carries out orders without any critical sense. He is the real zombie.

The poison was neither in Jacques's coffee, nor dispersed in his shoes, inside his clothing, or on the ground. He was gradually poisoned at his own workplace. The poison had been deposited on the armrest of his chair, and it penetrated the skin of his forearms each time that he sat down with his shirtsleeves rolled up, as he was accustomed to do. His mother-in-law used a middleman to deposit poison in the office, not taking the risk of doing the dirty work herself.

With his scientific perspective, Jacques still wonders how people who are "so little evolved" (*sic!*) could handle such a dangerous drug without poisoning themselves. "They say that tetrodotoxin is 100 times more powerful than cyanide. What manipulation enabled the production of the dosage necessary to make a man's life falter?"

As a clinical physician, Jacques Ravix is particularly skillful in describing the symptoms of his poisoning. He affirms that the initial sensation is that of a deep euphoria. Then, "you gradually withdraw into the night." At the end of a month of exposure, the first clinical signs have thus begun to appear. After the initial euphoria, a sort of insidious absence followed that worsened day by day. This did not impede him, however, from practicing medicine and seeing between twenty and forty patients daily, but he worked in a rather peculiar state all the same. Until one morning, he felt as if he were going to die, but "a quiet death," for the euphoria was still there. It was a euphoria "that carries one away."

His brother immediately came to get him to take him with all urgency to a *houngan* (Raymond Clavier), who they said knew how to treat this type of poisoning. Previously, this man had been a lawyer, but in the second half of his life he had taken on this responsibility as a Vodou priest. Jacques Ravix's feelings while his health was faltering, while he was losing consciousness and the antidotes were being administered to him, always remained positive. He felt well: "At least the experience was not unpleasant," he admits with a half-smile. It was as if a weight had left his body. At the end of a long ceremony, the *houngan* entrusted a vial of a product to Jacques' family that they had to administer to him by rubbing it on his body, but he added: "Be careful. You take a risk in treating him that the poison that infected him will also infect you." Furthermore, the product contained in the vial was not without its dangers. . . .

Once he had returned home, shortly after they had begun to spread this oil on his skin, Jacques Ravix fell into a sort of "coma." It was a very distinctive coma that he had never encountered in clinical practice, for he could still feed himself, dress himself, and do many things while being completely unconscious. It is what one calls total lethargy. His loved ones did not allow him to go out into the street. He could only walk around his bedroom or inside the house. He slept day and night, only awakening to eat. This state only lasted a few days before his full recovery.

For Jacques Ravix, it is because of the fact that tetrodotoxin is extracted from the liver of a scaleless fish (the Haitian *fufu* or Japanese *fugu*) that the Bible forbids the consumption of scaleless fish. When the *bokor* makes his zombie powder, he opens up this fish, retrieves the liver, and then leaves it to one side. But this is not all. It is also necessary to fetch a *bouga* toad that you introduce to a garter snake, and you provoke the toad "until he bursts with rage" . . . because he is scared to death of the garter snake. When it is dead, its venom is removed, which is mixed with the tetrodotoxin to obtain the active poison. Magical elements can also be added, such as the powder of human bones that are first scraped into shavings, but chemically they have no real effect. It is this toad venom that gives some victims extremely severe skin outbreaks of a very distinct kind. Other ingredients typically enter into the composition of *poudre à zombie*, such as millipedes, tarantulas, poisonous frog skin, roots, seeds of toxic plants, etc.

Tetrodotoxin destroys sensitive nerve fibers to such a degree that Jacques Ravix is now impervious to stings or small wounds. Some of his mucous membranes necrotized, particularly the end of his tongue, which he pulled from his mouth with his fingers (Jacques Ravix speaks of a "filthy, vile, stinking rot"). He has also suffered when it comes to his vision: his right visual field was reduced to such an extent that he no longer drives; over the course of his poisoning, he could not maintain distances with regard to other vehicles, and he caused fender-benders, if not serious accidents. Difficulty walking also set in, for his ligaments distended considerably, to such an extent that at the level of the hipbone, the head of the femur came out of the socket, causing a dislocation of the hip. He also developed anomalies of the liver and even the pancreas that rendered him diabetic. Not long ago, he had an electrocardiogram that showed the presence of a recent heart attack . . . but again, Jacques Ravix felt nothing. Is this linked to neurological desensitization due to the tetrodotoxin, or to the secondary effects of diabetic neuropathy? It is difficult to say.

Intellectually speaking, he lost his ability to concentrate for an extended period of time; forty consultations per day are now impossible. He cannot do more than five to seven in a row. If he still retains some sense, he no longer, on the other hand, has complete free will, and he sometimes adopts completely abnormal behaviors. Apart from within the professional setting, in which he functions "out of habit," he only does what he is told to do. It is impossible for him to say no.

If the drug had worked—in order words, if the appropriate dosage had been administered to him or if the *houngan* had not given him the antidote—Jacques Ravix is convinced that he would have been buried alive, and that the *bokor* hired by his mother-in-law would have come to get him and taken him from his grave right afterwards to turn him into a zombie with other spells and the help of middlemen and occult forces.

As a physician—and thus scientific and rational by nature—Jacques Ravix supports a very specific position with regard to this drug that changes the course of the life (and death) of men: "To awaken someone at the end of three days spent in an unopened casket is not possible," he says. "You need the help of a go-between, of entities that can work for the *bokor.*" His aborted zombification has made Jacques religious: "In the course of the rebellion of Lucifer (who became the fallen angel), some followed him, whereas others remained faithful to the Father. Those who followed Lucifer—the agents of Satan—spread out among men and did many evil things that only disappeared with the coming of Christ on Earth and his sacrifice." For Jacques, Vodou practitioners who make zombies are the descendants of these cursed beings, and he considers them to be Satanists (a tradition directly linked with Protestant churches, especially Pentecostal, to which Jacques Ravix does not, however, belong).

It is his way of healing. This experience has allowed him, in grazing death, to have a more intense religious life. Jacques thinks that God placed his hand upon him, and is protecting him from this point forward: "There is a certain comfort, but there is also anxiety. . . . Religious people are anguished because to discover another world, a parallel world, brings such dread, such anxiety that often, without the help of the divinity, it would be unbearable." Despite everything, he never complains. He knows what awaits him. Since he became a writer and a poet, it is in rhymes that he now sets his memories and hopes. His source of inspiration always remains his aborted death:

They are so beautiful, some days at the end of life.
When the homework is finished and the desks closed.
A child surprised by the rain runs toward the house
Where his father awaits him, standing in front of his door.
They are so beautiful, some days at the end of life.

CHAPTER 9

IN EROL'S PERISTYLE

Erol Josué's peristyle is not in the historic center of Port-au-Prince, but nestled in the working-class district of Martissant. To get there, you have to take one of these *tap-tap* (minibuses) covered with gaudy paintings, make it through the constant traffic jams, and, above all, you have to have patience. At the end of a tiny little street is a door of wrought iron decorated with the *vévé* (ritual drawing) of Baron Samedi. Behind, in the vegetation, hides the *hounfor* (Vodou temple) of this fascinating man. To the side, the peristyle has been freshly rebuilt after the earthquake of 2010. Covered with a concrete roof and quadrangular in shape, it meets earthquake-resistance standards—perhaps the only building in Haiti to do so! On the frescoes, partially repainted, it reads "Lafrique Guinin Society," a direct reference to this mythical land of Black Africa which slaves left from the 15th century onward, and where the souls of their descendants return after death.

Médor, Erol's dog—Erol must not have been very inspired at the time he named him—roams around the property, stretching out with a preference for the foot of the *potomitan* (or *poteau-mitan*) at the center of the peristyle. The *potomitan* depicts two green garter snakes in relief, intertwined like a caduceus (symbol of Damballa, the god of creativity, with his male and female parts), holding a white egg in their jaws (figure of life and of success). *Loas* take this pillar to descend to earth.

At first sight, one cannot really tell whether Erol (whom the daily newspaper *Libération* has nicknamed "Port of Prince Vodou"[1]) is a priest or a rock star, with his raspy voice, kinky red-dyed hair, intense black makeup around his eyes, and a disarming smile: today, he is wearing a skin-tight pair of dark jeans and a roomy Nirvana tee-shirt. This complete artist (he is also a singer and a dancer) has been stacking up cultural activities since the new president of the Republic of Haiti (Michel Martelly, himself a former popular singer) propelled him to director of the National Bureau of Ethnology (Bureau national d'ethnologie, BNE).

Inside Erol's peristyle, before drinking the coffee that he prepared, the master of the property gets up and goes to pour a few drops onto the four compass points at the foot of the *potomitan* as an offering to the *loas* before serving some to the living. In a corner, on a cane mat, there are ritual instruments half-covered with frayed, dusty fabric, including drums, drumsticks, and empty bottles ("It drinks a lot," like Erol says, without specifying whether he is speaking of the gods or the worshipers . . .).

Erol receives me in a wicker chair at the foot of the chamber of secrets in the back of the peristyle. Immediately, I ask him what is hidden behind the door. It is the altar of the *loas*, the place of mysteries, where the spirits reside and where worship instruments are stored, such as ornaments, dolls, statues, favorite beverages, pitchers, pre-Columbian stones (which represent the Taíno), machetes, accessories, etc. The entire history of Haiti is represented there. It is a sacred place of prayers and reflection where worship is led and then expressed around the potomitan at the center of the peristyle with the help of dances and chants.

Before returning to the chamber of secrets (*bagui*), Erol knocks (three times) to inform the *loas* of his arrival. Incidentally, in Haiti, when knocking on a door, it is customary to say "Honor," to which the host responds "Respect," before inviting the visitor to enter. Erol partially opens a door to his chamber of secrets. A scent made up of wet earth, spices, scented oils, dried blood, and alcohol escapes from it. It is a scent that I have smelled in the past in the private temples of the *bokonon* of Abomey in

Benin. While hanging out to one side (without entering, for I had not been invited inside by the *loas*), on an end table, I see some skulls, and a few long bones (tibias) hanging on the wall, those of the ancestors (blood or spiritual) who are such sources of inspiration.

There are three different mysteries, that is to say, three different places of residence of the spirits: those of the *loas* of Abomey (from Benin and the African continent in general), those of the Creole *loas*, and those of the *loas guédé* (the *loas* of the dead, generally at a distance from the peristyle in a separate small hut. Made entirely of concrete, Erol's is still under construction, and is awaiting its consecration in a few weeks). Adjacent to the peristyle, one finds the *lakou*, which reproduces, in small, the architectural and social organization of the African village (whose memory slaves have perpetuated). Small dwellings reserved for initiates (*hounsi*) follow one another in a semi-circle and, in the evening, each initiate meets up at the foot of the *potomitan* to share the story of the day and Vodou ceremonies. The deceased, problems, initiations, first communions (let us remember that Vodou practitioners go to church . . . perhaps also in order to provide a good education!), etc., give rhythm to these meetings.

Erol shows me around the property. The ground is wet; it rained during the night. A rooster wanders in the mud. Withered flowers fall with the morning wind. In the yard, I see orange peels hooked to the trees. Is this a magical practice? Not at all. Just a grandmother's household remedy for chasing away mosquitoes. This example brings to mind anthropologists' rule number one: Do not overinterpret.

Once again seated on the small wicker chairs, Erol Josué becomes loquacious about his religion and the attacks of which it is continuously victim on his native soil. The numerous churches present on Haitian soil lead to never-ending anti-Vodou campaigns: fourteen in total since 1804. The most significant one took place during the American occupation (1915–1934), another one during the 1960s,[2] and the last one after the departure of the Duvaliers (1986) during which 1,700 initiates were lynched and burned:

> All pastoral action of the Church in Haiti was organized in accordance with the struggle against Vodou. In fact, it is through this poorly

tolerated relationship that the Church has taken advantage of the legal framework in effect, particularly the statutory order of President Sténio Vincent dating from 1935 that resorted to the secular branch in 1940 and 1941 for the purpose of leading anti-superstition campaigns related to Vodou within the apostolic orientations. This statutory order was published on September 5, 1935. It is one of the documents of the Haitian State that informs the completion of all practical actions or others likely to maintain superstitious beliefs harmful to the reputation of the country.[3]

After the earthquake of 2010, some preachers also claimed that it was Vodou that had brought cholera. A veritable witch hunt followed, with a dozen *houngans* put to death by the mob. There was a new offense in July 2014 when Chibly Langlois (the very first Haitian cardinal) declared in an interview in the English newspaper *The Guardian* that Vodou is "a social problem . . . that will not save Haiti," pointing to the Vodou practitioners as "poorly educated." These remarks were immediately denounced by an interreligious group (including Catholics, Muslims, and Anglicans).

Not a day goes by without Christian churches accumulating anti-Vodou lectures. Some simulate cases of possession in which the victim claims "to have a *loa* in his head," "to be the devil," "to be Lucifer," and other grossly distorted folklores which, for Erol Josué, subjugate the people and continue to "zombify society," establishing a form of neocolonialism to which the churches that grow "like corn" on the island bear witness. It is thus that one of the major sites of Vodou history in Haiti (and also of the history of the nation itself) was hit head-on by this crisis of conscience. A tree had been planted by slaves in Bois-Caïman on the day of the ceremony of August 14, 1791. It was during this magical-religious ceremony that slaves gathered around *mambo* Cécile Fatiman drank the blood of a butchered black pig in order to make themselves invulnerable to the colonizers' bullets. This ceremony is at the origin of the insurrectional flame that ended in the creation of the Haitian state, simultaneously establishing Vodou as the protective religion of the revolution and then of the entire people. Yet this extremely symbolic tree was cut down a few years ago by Christian fanatics on the pretext that it "hosted the devil."

Then churches were constructed on the site in order to "decontaminate" it. Who gave the order for the desecration of this place, which, in addition to being a religious site, is a symbol of independence? A pastor, the grandson of a *houngan*. This represents a new "zombification of society" for Erol Josué, who appeals to a strong state to fight against this type of senseless destruction: "They do not come to evangelize, but to zombify. Missions arrive with their churches, their oils, their spoiled milk, and their rice. They brandish the Haitian flag while saying that it is the symbol of the devil. Haitians have no loss of identity, but rather an identity crisis caused by these people."

Yet the prayer of Dutty Boukman (one of the leaders of the Bois-Caïman ceremony) was an invocation of the Vodou gods (the *loas*), but also a text of profound tolerance that raises itself up against the colonizer's lack of understanding (and that of his god):

> The god who created the earth, who created the sun which gives us light.
> The god who holds back the oceans, who ensures the roaring of thunder.
> God who has ears to hear: you who are hidden in the clouds, who shows
>   us where we are, you see that the white man has made us suffer.
> The God of the white man asks him to commit crimes.
> But the God inside of us wants us to do good.
> Our God, who is so good, so just, commands us to avenge ourselves for
>   our wrongdoings.
> It is he who guides our weapons and who will bring us victory.
> It is he who will help us.
> We should reject the image of the god of the white man who is so
>   merciless.
> Listen to the voice of freedom that sings in all of our hearts.

In Port-au-Prince, a painting recently restored by France takes center stage in a room of honor in the Bank of the Republic of Haiti (*Le Serment des ancêtres* by Guillaume Guillon Lethière, 1822). This painting is one of the most significant symbols of the island and was taken charge of in Paris by the *Centre de recherche et de restauration des musées de France* (C2RMF) after the earthquake of 2010. In the painting are two slaves leaning on a headstone, praying for independence. God, depicted in the form of an old white man, overlooks them. The demon colonists have a hard life!

At the National Bureau of Ethnology (founded in 1934 in Port-au-Prince), Erol Josué responds point by point, and he proposes legislative advances to save the heritage and vibrancy of Vodou. Laws to protect the *loas*.

Erol Josué does not make zombies, but he knows this phenomenon well. In Haitian Vodou, it is the "secret societies" (Shampwel, Bizango, Zobop, Cochon gris, Secte rouge, etc.) that are responsible for this side, this dark, infernal side of the religion. Called "Vodou Tribunal" or "The Society," they operate and strike at night, judging individuals designated by their loved ones to be zombified or, to take back the common expression, "passed underground," or even killed. If Vodou decides to take charge of the matter, then they send a kidnapper to look for the individual, who is presented before the Society. They explain to him that he absolutely must change his behavior. They preach to him and then they judge him. Seven times in a row, this man "who prevents society from living" will be judged, and if he persists, then the secret society can decide that he cannot ultimately pursue his harmful action, and the society either zombifies him or kills him—by means of poison or a bloody death (provoked accident, forced suicide, simple assassination; all means are suitable). If a man is "too virile" and he harms the community, the Society castrates him, breaks him, and reduces him to nothing, as though it had physically said to him, "Calm down!" In other words, if he is not, purely and simply, put to death, then he may see himself suffer another form of existence, a "reduced life" such as a zombie life.

Secret societies traditionally originate from the indigenous army of Jean-Jacques Dessalines, which led the war of Haitian independence by fighting Napoleon's soldiers. It is a legitimate Vodou army that cannot be sees. It is not the official army, but it maintains the essence of its origins. It is an army that practices the justice that is specific to Vodou practitioners on the fringes of national laws, for "not everything that is legal is just," insists Erol Josué with an angelic look. In fact, he explains that followers of Vodou do not just pray, drink water, and dance. "Whoever can play the angel can play the devil," and sometimes action is necessary. After decades of colonization, Haiti lost nothing of its depths of superstitions and magical practices. After the death of Dessalines (1806), when the *repartimento* was brought about with the theft of territories in the mountains by varying armed factions, it was necessary for the Haitian people to bring justice when there was no Justice.

Even so, we must stop fantasizing. Zombies are not found on every street corner, just as they are not made in every *hounfor*. Even if they are part of daily life with this core of legends and magical-religious practices, zombies remain rare, and "it is not often that it works" (which means that errors in tetrodotoxin dosages are frequent and the victim is either only slightly ill or dies for good).

Erol Josué proclaims that he has never seen a zombie in his life ... but he believes in it, he knows that the zombie exists. He is not further tempted to see one, even out of the intellectual or professional curiosity of an ethnographer. He is not particularly afraid of them. Erol encounters other forms of zombies, Haitians who, because of what happens in their lives, are seen by others as zombies, yet they have never "passed underground." It might be severe depression, an individual who has been sent a *coup de mort* (in other words, whose soul was made ill by a potion administered by a *bokor*), etc. Erol has his own life philosophy, his own idea regarding the way in which he can avenge himself or seek revenge on others. He takes precautions in order not to be struck by magical spells. Therefore, he does not make zombies, nor does he promote zombies, but he understands very well why the zombie is important within secret societies.

While meeting the noise of the street again, I come to my senses. I am sure that Erol did not tell me the whole truth. But about what? Which secret(s) must he protect?

CHAPTER 10

ON THE TOMB OF NARCISSE . . .

The car speeds by outside of Port-au-Prince and drives along the sea to the lagoon waters. Source-Puante, Cabaret, Luly, Montrouis, Saint-Marc, Lafond, L'Estère . . . villages follow in succession as the light wanes. The sun is not far from setting when I arrive at the cemetery of Artibonite, a few kilometers from town. The place seems abandoned on the edge of the roadway. While the shadows grow, one hears the deafening sound of trucks loaded with merchandise that fly by at breakneck speed on National Highway #1.

I go forward into the cemetery while avoiding bones that litter the ground, including a child's mandible with its baby teeth, vertebrae of an elderly person deformed by osteoarthritis, foot and hand bones, etc. At the back of the cemetery, framed by old graves, is a concrete cross completely blackened with ashes and soot, as tall as a man. On the other side, engraved in the cement at the time of its construction, one reads the word "Baron." All around the cross, scattered on the ground in a complete shambles, are countless bottles of beer and rum that have been broken, offerings in calabashes (some pierced with holes) that have been burned (one of them still has a half-melted candle in the center of the hole), a cardboard box with chicken droppings and feathers spread out on the ground (connected to the animal sacrifices at this exact spot or to a simple meat offering to the *loa* that is then consumed by the believers: food for the gathering and for the gods), a head of a Barbie doll pulled from its torso (whose bleached-blond hair winds around the head three times and hides the face), clothing, and especially red or blue women's shawls, bits of rope, bottles of Pepsi, broken ceramics, candles that are not completely melted, oranges and a quantity of other fruits (now rotten), and numerous coins. In short, the devoted give food and drink, light candles, and scatter money in exchange for a service (healing, professional success, help with romance, etc.). In general, one does not ask Baron Samedi to cast spells, because he is a protector.

Baron Samedi is one of the forms of the Baron *loa*, along with Baron Cemetery or Baron the Cross. As a divinity of the dead, he is the spiritual father of the *guédés*. He is always dressed in black-and-white evening dress, a top hat, and sunglasses (one lens is broken), and his nostrils are plugged with cotton (like any corpse in order to avoid *post mortem* leakage). Quite free sexually, he excels in the *banda*, a very suggestive dance that imitates the act of reproduction. Each *loa* having his privileged time, such as Erzulie, who has her days (Tuesday and Thursday), Baron owes his name to the day of the week that is dedicated to him. Some invoke him to kill enemies or to bring a disobedient spouse to her knees (particularly at the precise moment of the dawn of the first Saturday in June), others to charm bees and guide them toward human targets to torture. His territory of preference is the cemetery, but he willingly accompanies souls of the dead on the road to Guinea, this mythical land of *post mortem* return to the African sources of transplanted slaves.

> It is a mythical place which, like the Christian heaven or paradise, would be a place where souls end up after death. When one dies, they say that one returns to Ginen by passing under the waters. In this specific instance, Ginen would designate the place of origin of the primordial ancestors, the place where souls reunite after death and settle down in a more or less permanent way on the primordial hill.[1]

The grave digger lives in the house next door along the road. Two young girls who are crossing through the cemetery to return home at the end of the night and to whom I explain that I am looking for the grave of Clairvius Narcisse hurry to go find the grave digger. Joseph Lixei is the name of this man. He is a round-shouldered old man who walks with a limp and is dressed in patched clothing, but he has a firm handshake and watchful eyes. His job as a grave digger in Estère consists only of putting the deceased in the ground. The family has to decide whether to add (or not, depending on their means or fears) cement to the tomb to make the potential removal of the body more difficult. What happens after the last shovelful of earth does not interest him. It is not part of his responsibilities. Besides, he leaves immediately afterwards. If loved ones want to make offerings, if they wish to come back to the gravesite, it is their business. "And what if someone (such as a *bokor*) comes during the night to unearth the body?" I ask him. He smiles (which is a way of saying, "It's fate"), but he does not answer. . . .

If, while digging a new grave, he ever comes across the remains of another deceased person, he gathers them and, without ceremony, he puts them back in the ground a short distance away. The grave digger explains to me that when families do not know exactly where the family gravesite is located (often because the unmaintained grave has been destroyed or reused), they come to bury their dead "near Baron." The place is considered not only protected (particularly against grave desecrators and *bokors*), but honored. From time to time, Vodou practitioners come to make offerings to Baron Samedi to ask for healing, success in love, or success on exams: "Baron is not only a protector. He heals everything."

Even if he is not a Vodou practitioner, the grave digger likewise makes offerings to Baron Samedi (not as a divinity, but rather as a patron, as if the god of the dead were his hierarchical superior, his *boss*). In Haiti, to make an offering is not necessarily a sign of allegiance or a mark of membership in one religion more than another. It is mainly linked to the fact that when one speaks to a divinity—no matter which—one must give it something in exchange for the expressed wish. Tit for tat. Such as when one goes to church gives to the collection during mass.

When the sun is touching the horizon, the grave digger finds the grave in a pile of undergrowth where he initially placed the body of Clairvius

Narcisse. It is a stone monument. Much of it is made of concrete, and it is completely ripped open. And with good reason, since a casket was dug up several decades ago that contained the body of a man who was still alive. Some rubble and wild grasses have since overrun this central cavity.

CHAPTER 11

PORT-AU-PRINCE, CAPITAL OF DEATH

The main cemetery is in the heart of the city, bordered by busy streets, the bus station, a soccer stadium, slums, and countless funeral homes. One enters it like going into a fortified castle, through a kind of drawbridge that spans a massive open-air sewer separating the world of the dead from that of the living. Just before crossing the high metal gates of the cemetery, a quote from Victor Hugo, painted on the wall in large, black letters, sets the scene:

I say that the tomb that closes upon the dead
Opens the heavens;
And that what we here below take for the end
Is the beginning.

On the ground, on the threshold, are chicken feathers, a lighted candle, and a few drops of blood. These are the remains of a Vodou ritual intended to protect equally the living from the evil dead and the dead from the living who are motivated by evil intentions.

The graves follow one another in a relatively normal way along the length of the main pathways, but on the side paths, everything becomes chaotic. Epitaphs are spread out, one after the other: "I am not dead. I have only left the earth in another life"; "Good soldiers die at home, said the Major to the deceased"; "The Eternal is great. Jesus is the savior of the world," etc. Nearly one hundred meters from the enormous entry, three crouching men dressed in black get up suddenly and scatter. I have hardly had time to witness their ritual. At their feet are a flaming calabash, a chicken whose blood escapes in gushes from its twisted neck, a few still-smoldering cigarettes, and a bottle of Barbancourt rum spilled on the ground. The offering has just taken place at the junction of the cemetery rows, the ideal place for the flow of mystical energies.

Since the work of William Seabrook, we know a few "recipes" used by *bokors* to make the dead come out of their graves (and then to make them return, lest they become too dangerous) or even to cast harmful spells. Let us judge the involvement of Catholic entities and divinities with Biblical or Near-Eastern connotations in these magical formulas and these diabolical rituals:

To evoke the Spirits. A Friday at midnight, meet at a road intersection. Obtain a candle made of fresh beeswax, beef fat, and swallow liver that you will light at this intersection in the name of Beelzebub while saying, "Beelzebub, I call you and I invoke you in order that you may reveal to me at this moment (such and such a thing . . .)." Next, you will fire a single shot, the weapon being loaded with incense and earth beforehand. Shoot toward the east while saying, "When the thunder rumbles, may all of the kings of the earth kneel down. May Puer, Agrippa Berke, and Astaroth spare me. Amen."

To evoke the dead. Go to the cemetery on a Friday night at midnight, carrying a white candle with you, a wild acacia leaf, and a loaded pistol, and choose the grave of a man. When you arrive there, you will say: "*Exurget mortui et acmo venient* (I demand that the dead man that you are come to me)." After having uttered these words, you will hear thunder. Do not fear anything, and fire a shot. The dead man will then appear. You must not flee, but back up three steps while repeating three times: "I spray you with incense and myrrh just as the tomb of Astaroth was perfumed."

How to send a Spirit back to the dead after having evoked it. Grab a handful of earth that you will throw to the four corners of the horizon while saying: "Return from whence you came, for you were created as dust and you will return to dust. Amen."

Blended with these curses focused on the deceased are other recipes with very practical connotations: how to create an invisible human figure, guard against bullets or torture, get out of prison, free yourself from a person who persecutes you, soothe a woman from the pains of childbearing, heal a sprained ankle, heal an injured eye, handle a toothache, rheumatism, yellow fever, etc. Performed in a context that is sometimes funereal and sometimes domestic, these rituals relate directly to the torments of daily life (contemporary to the 1920s, the time of their composition): illness, death, and the struggle against the Western oppressor.

Let us come back to the 21st century. In Port-au-Prince, the *bokor* who wishes to use human bones faces no major difficulties: when one wanders through the main cemetery, skeletons are everywhere. I only had to take the side paths and wander around between the plots to stumble across atlas moths, sacra, long bones, and mandibles. There were easily enough to piece together dozens of complete skeletons! There is nothing simpler for sorcerers. They go to the cemetery with a plastic shopping basket or a backpack, bend over discreetly, then leave once their crime is complete, the bag full of human bones, ready to be used. One literally walks on skeletons, just like on a carpet. Bones are everywhere: vertebrae, metatarsals, radiuses, and skulls. Children, adults, men, women: everything is, sometimes piled up in an ill-smelling heap. This flesh finishing its decomposition in the sun reminds me of the talisman markets of Abomey, Ouidah, or Cotonou (Benin)....

The earthquake of 2010 evidently accelerated the process, since many funeral monuments were ruined in the quake, or literally collapsed, pouring their contents into the pathways. But others were simply abandoned (the families sometimes died in the disaster, or they had other priorities than taking care of the long-deceased). In fact, many tombs are taken up by vagabonds who use them as a residence, or by other families who place their dead there after having emptied the initial contents and applied a coat of paint to erase any trace of the former owner. Others, out of a need for money, rent or sell a part of their plot. Of the four vaults that a tomb usually contains, two may be offered for rent—as stated on the banner adjacent to the name of the family of the deceased Fernand Gesner: "Two basement rooms at a firm price." There is practically a *post mortem* housing crisis.

On that day, I attend the funeral ceremonies of two men. The first was 55 years old. His family consists of about thirty individuals dressed to the nines in black or dark-colored party outfits and high-heels (15 cm high!) for the women. The Louis Vuitton bags have been dusted off. Loved ones are full of smiles, cheerful, particularly when bringing out the wreaths from the hearse and during the distribution of crowns and bouquets among the various relatives of the deceased. They joke, pull out flowers or plant them in their hair; photos or video are taken with cellphones. No sadness is visible in this procession that sloppily follows the white casket.

The second deceased person was 67 years of age. His family, all dressed in white and black, includes about fifty individuals varying in age from young children to old people. They sing the *Psalms of Praise* at the top of their voices with an undisguised joy from the street leading to the cemetery all of the way to the grave, while slowly following the spotlessly black hearse. Loved ones have smiles on their faces. It is more a party than a burial in the mournful and sad sense of the term. It is a celebration of the departed who is beginning his true life, the eternal one.

While strolling in the labyrinth of the muddy pathways that snake through the graves, I stumble across a monumental plot whose use was redirected in order to turn it into a Vodou temple. It is made of wrought iron, with angels on the four sides and crowns surrounding winged hourglasses. It is the grave of the Bienaimé Rivière family, whose name is still spread out in big letters along the façade, framed by the palms of martyrdom. The metal gate is closed with a padlock, and the interior is discernable only with difficulty behind plastic tarps and dark jute canvas extending the entire height. In the face of my curiosity, the *houngan* (Roland Gilles) allows me to enter. Inside, I discover a pigsty with numerous skulls, likely collected from neighboring graves, some of which are placed on red caskets with gilding containing names (Iazor, Florida . . .), religious statues (Christian—Saint Marguerite, Saint Expeditus, Saint Claire, a Black Virgin, Saint Martin, the Virgin Mary, Saint Blandine, etc.), bags wrapped in red fabric and tied up, plastic dolls with a cigarette in their mouths, numerous bottles of booze (some opened, and whose pungent scent climbs into the air), a small central altar made of marble (that of the Rivière family, whose name is still engraved on it) on which sits a skull with candles. They painted the name Marie on it (it is that of Marie Rivière, the first to have been buried in the monument and whose skeletal remains are bestowed with rather specific powers). On the table, I partially open a book with a faded cover: *L'Ange conducteur des âmes dévotes dans la voie de la perfection chrétienne* by Goret (Tours, Mame publishing, Editeurs Pontificaux). It is worn with use, and bears the trace of countless highlights. Scarves are hung on a metal bar behind an entry door (each with a different color corresponding to the *loas* to which they are dedicated: white for Damballa, purple and black for Baron Samedi and Dame Brigitte, blue for Erzulie Dantor, pink for Erzulie Freda, etc.). Right beside this, white underwear is drying. It contains nothing that is either religious or magical. It belongs to a *houngan*.

About fifteen yellowed, shriveled photographs are pinned up on the wall. Some are quite old, probably ten or twenty years old, judging by the clothing that the photographed subjects are wearing. Just as many followers have left a mark to ask the *loas* for protection: to heal an incurable or unidentified illness, to bring back an unfaithful husband, to make a marriage succeed, to save someone's job, etc. I am forbidden to touch the miniature caskets—red and black—that are piled up in a corner near the ground. Some have been there for a long time, as witnessed by the thick layer of dust and the rat droppings that largely cover them. "Too dangerous," the *houngan* says to me, "avoid even looking at them for too long."

The Vodou priest stores "magic" (types of mixes meant to bring luck and repel *coups de poudre* for which he holds the secret) in bottles of hair lotion (Aqua de Floride, Murray & Lanman, New York). He opens one of them and spreads the contents over my forearms and the palms of my hands. It is a citronella oil whose scent is very strong and a bit peppery. I do not know if this *eau de chance* protects against evil spells and poisons, but the experience has shown that it is a highly effective mosquito repellant!

East of the cemetery, not very far from the commemorative monument to the victims of the earthquake of 2010, rises a majestic tree twenty meters high. It stands among several graves, and a tiny courtyard has been installed on one side, like a kind of forecourt. It should be noted that this tree is a place of worship in and of itself, covered with Vodou dolls, bottles, wicker chairs, etc. According to the cemetery caretaker (Grégory Batau), *bokors* also come there to perform certain rituals and to place offerings when making zombies.

The bark nearly disappears behind the multitude of magical objects nailed to the trunk. Even the placement of the nail is not chosen by accident. For dolls, it is generally at the level of the heart, the head, or the pelvis, like so many anatomical targets. And when the nail rusts, the dolls fall from the tree and scatter on the top of neighboring graves and in the pathways. It is as if it were raining Vodou dolls.

The vast majority of dolls are single dolls. They are red in color, feature a human silhouette, and are filled with material and stitched on the sides. On the head and at the level of the pubis are also attached strands of hair from the head or body taken directly from the victim—in other words, the individual at whom the curse is directed. The *bokor* always obtains his supplies through go-betweens. Either the person who asks him for the spell collects these organic fragments from the target because he lives with him or her, or he pays the cleaning lady or the servant of the house so that in the early morning the said hairs can be taken from the bed of the future victim. Single dolls are for separate fates such as illness, death, loss of a trial, accident, etc. Double dolls, wrapped with wires or a padlock, are rarely red, but rather black and white, and are either for romantic purposes (to stir attraction and passion within the longed-for individual) or doubly evil (two people are targeted in the spell and linked in this curse).

I take advantage of the opportunity to collect seven of these Vodou dolls; they will pass over the balcony of my hotel room while waiting to be ritually deactivated. Once they are back in Paris, an X-ray exam shows the presence of objects belonging to the target in their filling (stuffing): a zipper, a button, etc. Others are punctured with countless needles. I counted up to one hundred of them on one of the double dolls!

On the tree, one notices stylized hanging ropes (the victim is willed to kill him- or herself or simply to die, no matter the means used, as long as the outcome is fatal), chairs on which dolls or objects belonging to the targets are tied together (a pair of black underwear, a pair of glasses, etc.), plastic bags with offerings (invisible from the outside) or hiding dolls on the inside, tracing paper on which a curse is written in Creole with magic signs, purple-colored fabric dedicated to Baron Samedi, etc. In areas that are hard to reach (one must climb on the adjacent tombs to reach them), candle fragments and chicken thighs bundled with black string are also hooked to the branches. Finally, at the foot of the tree is a crevice made in a fold of the trunk, partially closed by concrete blocks, in which a number of food offerings have been placed, primarily bottles of alcohol and . . . spaghetti with tomato sauce.

Several trees are growing in the cemetery. Why is this one the seat of such magical practices rather than another one? Those who are making offerings there tell me: "This tree has grown there since it was small. It has fed itself from the deceased people who surround it, who have decomposed and who form it. No one would dare cut down this tree, for a spirit (*loa*) protects it, and perhaps even numerous spirits." For others, the presence of a tree within a cemetery is unusual: "No one cut down this one because the spirit of a snake is inside it, and that keeps anyone from doing harm to it." This tree is magical. It serves not only as a zone of exchange between men and *loas*, but also, its touch can cause visions and make things that are distant in space and time visible as long as one makes an offering there.

It is a sacred tree. Upon taking a leaf from the tree to make a botanical identification, a *hounsi* tells me that I must toss a coin in the hollow of the trunk. Everything is a matter of exchange: "You take, you give. It is the law." The local name of this tree is *mapiang*, an epithet frequently associated with Erzulie, but its true Haitian name is *mapou*. It corresponds to the *Ceiba pentadra* (silk-cotton tree), a tropical and coastal tree of the Caribbean, Latin America, and West Africa. Considered sacred by the Taíno, they did not use its cotton (*kapok*) because they feared being possessed and suffering nightmares. For the Mayans, it is a *matou* that secured the axis of the world, and it is on it that the dead climbed to go from one celestial level to another. It is around the *mapou* that Vodou practitioners typically conduct their ceremonies, which take on an even greater power when the tree is located near a crossroads (meeting place for energies, site of the flow of *loas*). Children are usually told not to venture there at night because dangerous rituals—that they call "bloody" in order to frighten them—take place there at that time, right inside the trunk!

The cross of Baron Samedi is located near the wall of the cemetery. It is painted completely black, and is surrounded by a low wall that is also black, defining the zone of sacrifices; it is subjected to exceptionally frequent adoration rituals throughout the day. A wandering goat—quite fat—comes to nibble on the offerings placed by the faithful.

While I examine the empty bottles of alcohol left at the foot of the low wall, a plump woman suddenly emerges from between two plots and heads steadily toward the cross. She wears, thrown across her shoulders, a purple men's shirt (a color consecrated to this *loa*). Her eyes are rolled upwards (almost nothing but the whites are visible—how does she even walk?). She speaks a language that is not Creole—words of initiation?— addresses Baron Samedi, smacks the palm of her hands against the sides of the cross while going around it several times, rubs her own buttocks, thighs, breasts, and face (as if she were covering her own anatomical parts with particles from the cross), then leaves as slowly as she had arrived. Loved ones follow behind her at a reasonable distance, ready to intervene if her possession goes wrong.

A stone's throw away, Fanny, the *mambo* of Dame Brigitte, watches the scene with a disillusioned look. Seated on the stairs leading toward a monumental tomb, curvy, barefoot and in rags, her long pipe smoldering in her nearly toothless mouth, she has seen it all. Her territory borders that of Baron Samedi. It consists of a small esplanade painted all in white, with funereal *vévés* and a fresco depicting a marriage of skeletons drawn on the walls, framed with an inscription saying, "Happy birthday to all of the dead." In the center is a central altar set in the ground where several chicken carcasses are burning. In a corner, there are dozens of (empty) bottles of alcohol and a pair of high-heeled shoes (stilettos) attached to the grave next door, which serves as her house. Not very far away is an abandoned Vodou doll (swollen with water from the rains the night before) and two figures in grey and black fabric tied together with a string—obviously a love charm.

Antoine Sine, the man in charge of security in the cemetery, often sees strange things happen within the grounds of his workplace, especially at night. The weapon that he wears at his waist (a 9 mm) is there to prove that he is not here to goof around. Without being able to be more specific, he recounts that one evening he saw some people crouched on the ground in the process of performing "some kind of small ceremony." When he moved closer, these individuals fled on all fours like animals, then suddenly disappeared. A short while afterwards, Antoine was struck by fever, as if he had had to suffer their vengeance for having interrupted this important ritual. He then went to Léogâne to seek council and solace from the *houngan*, whom he knew, and that is the person who healed him. Since then, if Antoine comes across any *hounsi* or a *bokor* during the night, he does a U-turn. . . .

Patrick Scott, who is accompanying me in the cemetery, recounts a similar anecdote of an incident that happened in Port-Salut, along the southern coast of Haiti, at least twenty years ago. At the time, Patrick was interested in this area because there was a truly magnificent little beach there: it was an old disused landing strip turned back into a field that descended gently to the sea. So he was heading toward this cove and, when almost halfway there, he came across someone he did not know. (Patrick smiles as if to protect himself from recounting something so huge.) It was a man between 30 and 40 years old with a strange, tough look (a look that Patrick had already seen during Vodou ceremonies), evil, full of reproach, as if he were saying to him, "What are *you* doing here?" And at the moment when he turned around Patrick witnessed this man transform into a steer. He began to walk differently. His body was altered. "Suddenly, he was no longer a man." He must have been on a mission, but he was not necessarily a *houngan* or a *bokor*. "There are people here who have powers. Powers that were granted by gods. Their own gods."

CHAPTER 12

ZOMBIES AT THE COURTHOUSE

Emmanuel Jeanty is a criminal-law attorney at the Cap-Haitian bar. I meet him at the Court of Appeals of Port-au-Prince, a collection of prefabricated buildings in which the Haitian justice system has reorganized itself since the earthquake of 2010. A graduation ceremony is taking place outside, under a tent. An entire group of judges in ceremonial clothing gathers to hear a minister give his speech. In the small hall, which smells like freshly cut wood, Maître Jeanty sits down on a corner of a desk and raises his voice a bit as if he were pleading a case.

Nearly every day, if one believes Haitian radio or television, there is talk of deceased residents whose funeral ceremonies have taken place who then, a short while afterwards, have been found alive. Or of *bokors* who die and at whose home is discovered a hut in the courtyard sheltering a dozen zombies. According to Jeanty, these accumulated cases end up creating problems at the very heart of society, which drove him to address the cases of these zombies legally. His concern is very ordinary: What does one do with the debts left by this undead individual? How does one manage his estate, since he is not truly deceased? What is to be done with his property? Is it given back to him, or left with his heirs? How does one restore a legal existence to an individual declared dead, for whom accounts have been closed, his passport shredded, and the death certificate signed? Haitian legislation does not recognize zombies, since to exist legally, a person must at least have a birth certificate. The zombie being a subject who is falsely declared dead, it is impossible, as it stands at the moment, to turn back. One cannot establish either a "rebirth certificate" or a "confirmation certificate of erroneous death." The zombie has no legal existence and no nationality. He is no longer anything (and that is exactly what *bokors* are seeking to create).

Until now, no "certificate of resurrection" has been proposed in Haitian legislation. Nevertheless, Clairvius Narcisse's case served as a catalyst for sorting this out. He traveled abroad, got remarried, and had children. Any travel outside of the territory requires a declaration, just as any birth requires the citizen to report the new child and the name of its father . . . in theory.

The majority of Haitian judges maintain that cases of zombification are not specified in the legislative and judiciary systems of the Republic. Maître Jeanty thinks the opposite. Article 246 of the Haitian Penal Code, in fact, does not recognize the status of zombie (the word does not appear there), but a "state of lethargy." Is this sufficient? Rather often in Haiti, people say that there is no legal provision to judge an individual for zombification. Yet Maître Jeanty conducted an analysis based on the fact that the code used in Haiti was adopted in 1835 and is inspired by the Napoleonic Codes. By deciding to accept this legislation that came from another country, the Haitian people have, *ipso facto*, also imported onto the island all of the problems, strategies, and aspirations that ravaged France during this era.

Does this mean that the phenomenon of zombies also existed in Europe during the first half of the 20th century? Not exactly. But since the 17th century, a considerable number of works on the undead and unjustified burials have appeared. The most famous are *De la mastication des morts dans les tombeaux* by Michaël Ranft (1725), *Traité sur l'incertitude des causes de la mort, et l'abus des enterrements et embaumements précipités* by Jean-Jacques Bruhier d'Ablaincourt (Paris, 1742), and *Traité sur les apparitions des esprits et sur les vampires, ou les revenants de Hongrie, de Moravie, etc.* by Lorrain dom Calmet (Paris, 1746). These were true bestsellers that spread the idea that it was possible—and even common—to be buried alive. These collections of anecdotes were so widely spread throughout Europe and the colonies that they influenced minds to the point of even modifying burial systems[1] and introducing the use of specific instruments to verify the absence of signs of life at the moment the corpse was into the coffin (a silver needle forced under the nail of the big toe while watching for a possible reaction to the pain; cutting a vein or an artery to verify the absence of blood flow, etc.). Some cases described by authors, in fact, speak of "dead who chew" or of others who tried to get themselves out of their coffins by scratching the wood on the inside or who ate their own fingers because they were so hungry or thirsty before finally dying. Other examples—this time, literary—exist, such as in Shakespeare's *Romeo and Juliet*, *The Count of Monte-Cristo* by Alexandre Dumas (Edmond Dantès), or even *Hadriana dans tous mes rêves* by René Depestre. Zombies obey what appears to be a universal reality.

As evidence, these recent cases typically make the headlines because they respond to an age-old question (and a fear). In 2014, the heart of an American woman, victim of an amniotic embolism during childbirth, stops beating for 45 minutes, and starts up again just before the physician pronounces death. A Polish woman, 91 years of age, is declared dead and regains consciousness at the morgue . . . and even a doctor, Anna Bagenholm, fell into icy waters during a hike and survived nearly an hour of asphyxia.[2]

Throughout my career as a forensic pathologist, I recall having faced situations such as these on two prior occasions. In the first case, a woman had made a suicide attempt with the help of drugs that slowed down the heartbeat (beta blockers) and had been found, apparently dead, by her cleaning lady at her home. The word "deceased" having been pronounced from the onset, the emergency physician simply signed the death certificate, then the body had been photographed by the police and moved by the funeral home to the refrigerators of the morgue where she ended up dying from hypothermia. In the second case, an elderly woman, similarly, was pronounced dead prematurely, but her loved ones realized their error while removing her jewelry in the body bag. Immediately transported to intensive care, she ended up dying three days later from a massive stroke.

Article 246 of the Haitian Penal Code mentions the following:

Is considered poisoning, any attempt on the life of a person through the use of substances which can cause death more or less quickly, regardless of the manner in which these substances were used or administered, and regardless of the consequences.

It does not matter whether the poison was placed in fruit juice, water or any other drink, in his or her food, shoe, or clothing, without the victim's knowledge. It does not matter whether it acted as an ingested liquid or as a powder spread on the skin. It does not matter what process was used to administer the *coup de poudre*. Let us consider Article 246 again:

Is also considered an attempt on the life of a person, by poisoning, the use made against a person of substances which, without causing death, will produce a more-or-less prolonged state of lethargy, regardless of the manner in which these substances were used and regardless of the consequences. If the person was buried as a consequence of this state of lethargy, the attempt will be considered a murder.[3]

As Maître Jeanty cites:

As a precaution, the victim called to become a zombie must inevitably go the mortuary route in order that his executioner might avoid being arrested for illegal confinement or abduction (kidnapping). Moreover, Article 306 of the *Penal Code* forbids the violation of graves and additionally prescribes: "Will be punished with imprisonment from three months to one year whosoever will be found guilty of tomb or grave violation, without prejudice against crimes or misdemeanors that would be combined with this." Thus, even when it is insufficient, there are still a few related texts, even when the term *zombification* is not expressly used.[4]

We still must wonder how it is possible to bury a "powdered" individual in a lethargic state while being unaware that he is, in fact, still alive. The answer is perhaps hidden in the Haitian Civil Code, particularly Article 77, which focuses on deeds and documents:

The death certificate will be made out by the state registrar upon the testimony of two witnesses. If it is possible, these witnesses will be the two closest relatives or neighbors, or when an individual will have died outside of his home, the person at whose home he has died, and a relative or another individual.

In other words, in order to pronounce a death, two witnesses suffice. It is not necessary to have the body examined medically, which opens the door to many irregularities. The registrar requests no medical or scientific justification regarding the condition of death of the subject. Two members of a family wishing to get rid of an annoying relative can thus "powder" him with the help of a *bokor*, then falsely declare their relative dead and turn him into a zombie without being troubled by anyone.

This article, like the rest of the Haitian Civil Code, was adopted in 1826! If one can understand that in the first half of the 19th century, the number of physicians was sufficiently low for it to be necessary to go through them to declare someone deceased, it is possible to say that the situation has in all likelihood changed at the beginning of the 21st century. A new medical specialty appeared (forensic pathology), and others came to supplement the field of possibilities, permitting—theoretically—the diagnosis of death with some certainty: anesthesiology, resuscitation, toxicology. In fact, there are numerous circumstances placing an individual in a state of apparent death in such a way that he might be considered dead by those around him while his vital functions are only slowed down: ingestion of toxins (apart from tetrodotoxin, one must include beta blockers—medications that reduce blood pressure and heart rhythm—and barbiturates), metabolic disorders (severe hypoglycemia, hypothyroidism), hypothermia, locked-in syndrome (or brainstem stroke, an illness described in detail by Jean-Dominique Bauby in his autobiography, *The Diving Bell and the Butterfly*), and psychiatric disorders such as necromimia in which some patients "play dead."

In Haiti today, they can no longer afford to leave care to just anyone—in other words, to people who have not studied medicine and who have no experience in the precise diagnosis of death necessary to pronounce a death definitively. Perhaps Article 77 should be modified with the goal of modeling advances in scientific knowledge and the modernization of medical practices? Yet funerals can take place only after 24 hours have passed since death (in theory, to allow time for signs of death to appear: rigor mortis and lividity).

The Haitian Criminal Code of Instruction (law of July 30, 1835, Article 34), the equivalent of France's Penal Procedural Code, specifies the conditions in which dead bodies must be examined:

> If it is a case of a violent death or a death whose cause is unknown or suspect, the Government commissioner will have one or two physicians, surgeons, or healthcare officers create their report on the causes of death and the state of the victim's body.

If one draws from the work completed by ethnobotanist Wade Davis—especially his use of tetrodotoxin on some subjects—what should a doctor in Haiti do to assure a "real and permanent" death? Use specific tools such as a stethoscope or a sphygmomanometer (to take blood pressure). Another possibility would be to wait for indisputable signs of death before diagnosing death then proceeding to funeral preparations: lividity, rigor mortis, protruding blisters, green abdominal blemish, etc. Most often, in Haiti, the registration of death with the state registrar takes place without delay right after the individual has passed away (as they say, "on a body that is still warm").

To this strict deadline and to the skill of the observer must be added the suitability of tools used for the diagnosis of death. Can simple clinical inspection—sometimes swift—combined with a cardiopulmonary auscultation eliminate the possibility of a state of apparent death? Not always. It is sometimes necessary to conduct additional examinations to avoid a misdiagnosis because these tools are not suitable for cases of zombification. If one believes Maître Jeanty, it might, perhaps, be necessary to create special biomedical teams responsible for testing zombies at the time of administrative declarations of death in the event of a suspicious death. The only problem with this is that nearly all deaths in Haiti are suspicious. . . . If there is any doubt, the family or beneficiaries could call in specialists to detect whether the individual is under the influence of zombification, even ask a *houngan* to lend them a hand, or a council of *houngan* to issue a guide of best practices or conduct a meeting of consensus with the goal of defining reliable and detectable zombification criteria. On the criminal level, the implementation of systematic tests could be set up in the same way, within the obvious limits of the finances of the implicated government departments (Justice and Interior).

For Maître Jeanty, given that the problem of zombies has become specifically Haitian, civil and penal laws regarding death must also be Haitian, free of European influences that no longer have any practical justification in the current chrono-cultural context. They must be focused on their own problems and their own characteristics in order to be more effective and more viable.

This lawyer's work is focused on a proposition of advancements regarding criminal legislation. But he is also interested civilly in the recognition of those for whom zombification has already taken place, those who wander between two worlds and who are no longer anything at the administrative level. For their defense, Maître Jeanty thinks that using the *Universal Declaration of the Rights of Man* (1948) can be justified. The preamble states the following: "The recognition of the inherent dignity and of the equal and inalienable rights of all members of the human family is the foundation of freedom, justice and peace in the world." What can legislation thus do for the recognition of someone who is "dead" under conditions that are found on the margins of science (in other words, neither explained nor clarified), and who then resurfaces? Is it necessary to have a trial to have the person recognized as alive again? If the zombie causes a problem to a third party, to whom—which entity—will the latter be able to turn? The state? The zombie's former parents? The zombie himself (difficult, given that he was declared dead and no longer has any legal existence)? Upon arrival at court, any zombie accompanied by a good lawyer would hold his death certificate in his hand, saying: "Look. I am dead. I thus cannot be held accountable for anything." Why would the responsible party not then be the *bokor*, the sorcerer who zombified him? But then, that would necessitate both another police inquiry and another scientific investigation that makes the link between the medical history of the patient who became a zombie and the materials found at the home of the *bokor*.

Here in Haiti, Maître Jeanty is a Don Quixote. He conducts all of his travels at his own expense because the subject interests him considerably. His work extends to the national level, and he is beginning to hit the mark with the Ministry of Justice: a reform or, at least, a reworking of the laws is in progress, a sort of weeding out of texts that are too old simply to be slightly updated. Will Maître Jeanty's law colleagues bring new legal initiatives from foreign countries? The problem is that some suspicions are specific to Haitians, and that Western law is not entirely suitable. In France (just as in the United States, Italy, Germany, etc.), when an individual is suddenly found dead in his bed, it is the responsibility of the medical examiner to determine the causes and circumstances of death. In Haiti, priority is given to funeral plans without worrying about determining the specific cause of death and without always suggesting that an investigation be opened. Is this deliberate?

Whether real or fake, not a year goes by without a zombie case surfacing. Sometimes, a *bokor* is suddenly dead in the countryside, and when dealing with his estate it is discovered that he had a little house in the courtyard of his home that lodged zombies. And since this master is dead—that is, their executioner or kidnapper—it is as if the zombies are freed, and they meet to wander aimlessly in the streets or in the markets. In general, nobody worries about these individuals, except when they have the chance of being recognized by loved ones who thought they had been dead and buried long before. But in legal terms, they have no existence. Anyone can hit them, beat them up, and abuse them, and will not incur any punishment, since the victim has no "stability" in legal terms. The zombie cannot even be called a person, since he no longer has either a birth certificate or an identity. In fact, there is actually no legislative text recognizing zombies as individuals. Much more than a question of semantics, it is a question of the restoration of rights lost through a magical action. The law does not recognize anyone if he or she does not have a legal existence, in the same way that slaves were not recognized as human subjects during the triangular trade, but rather as animals or chattel. Legal texts in Haiti that address the cases of these people are thus necessary, perhaps resulting in a "Jeanty Law" that finally recognizes the very specific status of these individuals living between two worlds.

Haitian culture is a breeding ground of options as much for the social as for the religious emergence of zombies. To create a zombie is to escape traditional justice. To make a zombie is to carry out a sentence that is worse than death. It is to make someone live his own death and then to keep him alive while at the same time depriving him of his own will. It is to transform him into a modern-day slave, but also to remove from him all critical sense, all accountability, and all humanity.

According to Maître Jeanty, Haitians are reluctant, at first glance, to call in a medical examiner—even if one bears in mind that in this area, like all those of African tradition, nearly all deaths are suspicious: "They always believe that if the individual underwent a zombification ceremony, then the physician will kill the *bokor*'s victim once and for all while performing the autopsy, and that will be it for the person." This is an erroneous idea, of course, for the practitioner obviously makes sure that the patient he must dissect is really dead—and no matter what, he would be aware of it through a pulsatile flow of blood at the first cut of the scalpel. But not all Haitian doctors are technologically able to detect cases of zombification. A simple clinical examination neither systematically nor easily enables it. Infrequent and very low-intensity heartbeats are not necessarily palpable either to the pulse or to auscultation, depending on the positioning of the body, the conditions of the examination, and the body weight of the subject. Maître Jeanty calls for the bringing in of the appropriate diagnostics to Haiti.

In Haiti, there are only two medical examiners for ten million citizens. Despite the creation in 1999 of Uramel (*Unité de recherche et d'action en médecine légale*, whose mission is the promotion of forensic pathology and health rights to all parties involved in Haitian life[5]) by one of the examiners (Dr. Jeanne Marjorie Joseph, trained at Université de Rennes), forensic autopsies are rarities in this country. When a body is found in the street or when a murder takes place, a simple external examination (with no autopsy) is performed by a physician after the body is transported to the hospital. Why? In all likelihood, it is because no practitioner wants to take on this area specialty—that of opening corpses for the Ministry of Justice. Unless it is about nothing more than a fear specific to the judge himself?

Judges are not authorized to pronounce a death officially (except when it is obvious: a severed head at a distance from the body, or a completely rotted, burned, or skeletonized corpse, for example). They are required to rely on either a partial administrative process (declaration of death by two witnesses who can present a significant conflict of interest) or a medical examination completed without modern means of screening for states of apparent death. Maître Jeanty is almost at the point of asking for (or hoping for) a systematic dosage of tetrodotoxin for each Haitian "corpse," a team of scientific specialists, and technological tools suitable for screening zombies. "We could have some surprises!" He is even proposing that an association of *houngans* be available to adjudicate in cases in which there is any doubt regarding the true nature of a death or zombification. This is a solution that would certainly not please *bokors*—and we are aware of the risks involved in opposing their power. Just as medical examiners take an oath "to provide support for Justice honorably and in good conscience," why not do the same with *houngans*, he says, by making them swear (on the Haitian Penal Code or on the Bible?) to engage in establishing the truth? The ideal would be to turn a *bokor* away from the dark side (black magic) to which he consecrates his magical-religious activities. For Maître Jeanty, this does not seem impossible.

The *houngan* in Haiti, this "connoisseur in the field of leaves," is often seen as a doctor, and therefore consulted by patients who cannot travel to a clinic or who can pay neither for short-term hospitalization nor surgery. This healer—in the broadest sense of the term—can achieve an equivalent of a doctor's certificate, which Maître Jeanty calls a "*hounfor's* certificate," in other words, a certificate established in the field of his own expertise, which is magical-religious practices. The official recognition of these practices already takes place at the highest level of the Haitian state (even indirectly), as leading politicians travel as far as Artibonite to have their neurological illnesses cared for by renowned *houngans*.

Second, the *houngan* is also seen as a soothsayer, a seer, a man who knows from where evil comes, but equally as an adviser in the countryside; he can become a *bokor* when he makes ill-advised use of magical processes (to do wrong, to curse, to kill, or to zombify), like a being with split personalities, twin abilities, and dual power. But not all *houngans* have this dark side, and Maître Jeanty is certain that the majority of them will take an oath before the country's justice system to counter the effects caused by *bokors*, like in a Manichaean struggle between good and evil. When he is told that this image puts one in mind of Harry Potter a bit, he smiles as well, but he is firmly convinced of it. "We are not talking about magic wands here, nor about brooms that fly. It concerns men buried alive in caskets from which they must be removed before they are completely dead or tested before they are put underground."

The phenomenon of zombies has inspired many scientists, including the least honest and the most audacious. Some, in fact, intend to use zombification as an experimental practice designed to heal illnesses deemed grave and incurable, such as diabetes or HIV infection. In their work (especially controversial and, quite obviously, certainly not recognized by the international community), they actually claim that that some subjects suffering from these illnesses were involuntarily "whitened" (in other words, "healed" or "made better") after their poisoning by tetrodotoxin. Are we not, here, in the territory of a myth of rebirth similar to the fantasy of the fountain of youth from which the souls of the dead drink during their underground stay? "It is a question of old data, and it is necessary to test this working hypothesis scientifically on current subjects. Alas, we are lacking volunteers," Maître Jeanty adds with irony.

But, as we have seen, the term zombie can encompass very different realities: the "true" zombie, the fruit of toxicological and magical practices; a zombie of a social nature (with a more or less voluntary change of identity facilitated by a real problem involving identity and the handling of personal records in Haiti); and, finally, the zombie with a nearly psychiatric connotation (pathomimia, necromimia, multiple personalities, and especially the individual who has known death).

Why does the zombie exist? For Maître Jeanty, the zombie as a social phenomenon responding to an identity crisis does not explain everything. To the Gonaïves in Cap-Haïtien towards Jacmel, in Saint-Louis-du-Sud, there are multiple cases of individuals who passed from life to death and who are then seen again, safe and sound. According to Maître Jeanty, these are too numerous to be a simple perversion of the system for the purposes of social escape. Clairvius Narcisse's case is perhaps the most media-friendly, and the most exploited, scientifically speaking. But that of Natagete Joseph in the 1960s-1970s is also particularly instructive. The lawyer, who is greatly interested in symbols and in spirituality, did not hesitate to go up and down the entire island to document cases of zombies as much as possible, but also to question *bokors* in order to "squeeze things out of them." He was unsuccessful. Due to lack of an initiate (*hounsi*), it was impossible to obtain information on their *modus operandi*—at least more information than Wade Davis had obtained in the 1980s.

Does Maître Jeanty fear either *houngans* or *bokors*? "Definitely not," he answers without hesitation. In Haiti, justice is not often served as it should be. If something happens to him one day, Maître Jeanty will likely see justice done because he knows his rights, because he is part of one of the largest law offices in the Republic, and because he is a consultant and a professor at the university. But this justice is not divided homogeneously on the island, and this heterogeneity digs the *bokors*' bed of power. Maître Jeanty studied their way of being, of speaking, and of working. He knows them better than anyone. Whether or not one believes it, anyone can be touched by a *coup de poudre* because it is "chemical" well before it becomes spiritual. It is a matter of only a few milligrams deposited in a shoe or on clothing. How does one fight against it? It does not matter whether one is Catholic, Protestant, Muslim, a Freemason, or agnostic. Nothing will make any difference. Nothing will prevent the poison's harmful action on the human body. Nothing will resist the poisoning. The case is similar to a loaded pistol pointed right at the victim: the shot will leave at all events as soon as the trigger is pulled, no matter what the victim's convictions might be.

Maître Jeanty was introduced to the general public through a particularly media-friendly forensic case involving a man living in the Dominican Republic as a *braseros* (itinerant worker), but who, like his parents, he was serving the *loas*. One fine day, his wife called him on her cell phone to tell him that if he did not return to Haiti, a tragedy was going to occur: "There is a werewolf (a type of *macanda*) that wants to remove the souls of our two children." The man thus bought a dagger in the Dominican Republic, conducted a ceremony over there, then returned home and lived for two months without seeing either the slightest demonic manifestation or apparition. Then, he took a bit of rice and began to prepare his return trip to the Dominican Republic. But during the course of that same evening, he suddenly heard a sound in the courtyard, and when he came out, he saw a strange animal that had the colors and the appearance of a tiger and a dog. The man immediately attacked the animal with his dagger. Wounded, it fled and crossed over a small hedge to end up in the neighboring house, that of the man's father. Dagger strikes followed each other, then the animal transformed into a human being—the father of the accused—who allegedly said in Creole: "This is going to be the end of me."

If the story sounds like a real fairy tale, it has nonetheless been pleaded in circuit court as an assassination and parricide (December 2008), and Maître Jeanty, on the side of the defense, won the trial (which was filmed in its entirety). If, according to Article 247, the Haitian Penal Code stipulates that parricide is never justifiable, Maître Jeanty succeeded in creating a precedent, since, in the present instance, he succeeded in having a legitimate excuse recognized. He did not, however, base his plea on the use of poisons or drugs that would have clouded the judgment of the accused, but he founded it rather on the "culture," to use one of his own terms. This man had the house of his father—who had little means by which to live—rebuilt, he looked after him, gave him signs of affection, of filial piety, bought him clothing, and did not stop sending him money from the Dominican Republic. Why, therefore, would he have killed his father?

Maître Jeanty has not yet pleaded any zombie cases, but, just as he says himself, he "cannot wait." . . . Now, he is ready.

CHAPTER 13

LODGE OF THE ZOMBIES

Dr. Girard practices at the psychiatric hospital of Port-au-Prince. His office opens in a small street-level building in the main courtyard of the establishment. On the walls hang his foreign diplomas, photographs, and drawings made by some of his patients. His medical books, some specialized magazines, and countless medical files are piled up in the cabinets. In the air, the unbearable whirling of mosquitoes and Creole music radiates from the outside (from street vendors of cassettes and CDs). The doppelganger of Morgan Freeman, Dr. Girard exudes benevolence. Not a Vodou practitioner himself, for several years he has been in charge of a patient considered to be a zombie.

This woman (Adeline D.) was pronounced dead at two o'clock in the morning of July 25, 2007, aged just forty. Drafted in the town of Limonade and signed by two witnesses—her sister, Marie D., and a cousin named Destouches—her death certificate bears witness to this fact. Several deaths had occurred around her shortly beforehand, four nearly simultaneously (including her father, her mother, and a sister). Before her funeral ceremony, the body remained approximately three days in the morgue, then Adeline D. was placed in the freshly cleaned vault. But at the time of the burial, the grave digger began to put financial pressure on the family. No mortar or cement had been purchased, and long debates began on the subject of the right sum of money to pay. Discouraged, around 4:00 or 5:00 p.m., when it was almost night, the loved ones left the corpse in the vault without ensuring that the hole was correctly sealed, and returned home.

Adeline D. was discovered by her sister (a nun), completely by chance, around one year after her official "death." The encounter occurred near a seminary in Cap-Haïtien, about thirty kilometers from her cemetery. Adeline D. was wandering in the street, haggard, her hair shaven, emaciated. Her sister immediately led her to the Catholic priests to undergo an exorcism (it was unsuccessful). A short while later, her sister being a superior in the congregation of the Daughters of Mary, she brought Adeline D. with her to Port-au-Prince. There, in a small shack, in rags, hair cut short, still in the same clothes (pink T-shirt, green skirt, broken sandals), a rosary around her right wrist and very thin, Adeline D. survived miserably by doing basketwork. Having become the patient of Dr. Girard in November 2013 (the date of her hospitalization at the psychiatric center), she still refuses to wash herself and to change clothes.

Adeline D. thus spent between nine and twelve months in a semi-conscious state in the service of others. How was she able to leave her zombie condition? One day, she went to look for bread, and there was a fight. She fled and ended up near Sainte-Thérèse seminary in Cap-Haïtien where, three months later, her sister had found her. Adeline D. then disappeared again for several months before she reappeared and was brought to Port-au-Prince. Other zombies were freed during the earthquake of 2010 when their "masters" were killed in the collapse of homes.

Obviously, Dr. Girard wanted to verify Adeline D.'s identity by comparing her DNA with that of her close relatives. She had previously had four children (one died, and among the three survivors was a set of twins). The results were problematic. Not only do the twins (a boy and a girl named Cathelin and Catheline) not have any genetic link to Adeline D., but it also seems that they have no direct link to each other! Everything is complicated in Haiti. It is said that the civil registry is rather poorly maintained, and numerous adoptions are unreported—to say nothing of cases of adultery. . . . Actually, these results are not necessarily interpretable and do not make it possible to rule out this woman as being Adeline D., dead and buried on July 25, 2007. Dr. Girard thus hopes to go to Limonade as soon as possible to verify whether or not there is a body in this vault and, if human remains are still present, to identify this corpse genetically by comparing the results with those of other members of the family (ideally, her sisters).

Dr. Girard brings me to visit Adeline D. in her room—or rather, her cell. She is hospitalized voluntarily here—in other words, she is authorized to leave during the day, but must return to her room before nightfall. We stroll in the gardens, passing in front of a poorly maintained official plaque: "This lodge was constructed with the generous contribution of His Excellency Mr. Jean-Claude Duvalier, President of Haiti for life, Mrs. Simone O. Duvalier, First Lady of the Republic, the Baroness Nicole de Montesquiou Ferenza, Dr. Nathan Kline, and the National League for Mental Health."

A hallway sinks into the depths of the main building. In one corner, rusted iron gates seal off a gloomy recess. My colleague calls the patient, who gets up from her mat and, groping around in the darkness, finds her key, opens the gate, and turns on the light. The single bulb, at the center of the room, illuminates in a pale light a completely unlikely outpost.

In a corner, a mattress placed on the ground serves as her bed and desk. Her papers are thrown on the sheets and the blanket with some pens, pencils, and a few brochures. On the opposite side of the room and in an adjoining nook, numerous plastic bottles are piled up. Adeline D. drools a lot, and always walks with one of those bottles to spit into. For Dr. Girard, if one does survive this poisoning, hypersalivation is one of the secondary signs of tetrodotoxin intoxication, and can become chronic or sequellary.

On all of the walls of the hospital, Adeline D. has drawn the *vévés* of Baron Samedi and Dame Brigitte with charcoal, but she has also drawn phalluses, knives, sabers, etc. When I ask her why, she explains to me that she was invited to dinner with them during her brief stay underground and they taught her these symbols. Almost no wall escapes the Kabbalistic signs left by this patient, beginning with her cell, of course, and all the way to the exterior doors of the psychiatric hospital, as if she had wanted to set up a circle of protection around herself or to consecrate this place to the gods of the dead.

She only draws on the walls. Entire pages are scrawled with her cross-words, her vague calculations, her incomprehensible symbols, and with several portraits.

Dr. Girard has snapshots of his patient before her "death." She was tall and slender, smiling, and rather pretty. Since her hospitalization, she has gained weight. She cuts her own hair from time to time, and she always wears black. Her days are extremely ritualized. She goes out every morning at 8:00, spends her time in the park, then she returns every evening at 5:00. Each morning, she eats the same seven very specific foods (including bread, spaghetti, figs, and blackberries) whose arrangement on the ground is formulaic.

When she was in a state of zombification and reduced to slave conditions at home, she took care of two children (Melita and Melissa). Her masters gave her a new name (Mirlande Antoine) and a common nickname (*Ti Momi*). This change of identity is one of the major signs of the social phenomenon of zombification. Adeline D. frequently draws the house in which she stayed and worked while she was a zombie. It is a four-story building with the kitchen downstairs, the dining room on the main floor, the living room on the second floor, then a living room/bedroom on the top floor. Framing this design are people (two adults and two children) with neither arms nor ears, a direct sign of the absence of the physical contact that she had with them; to touch a zombie brings bad luck, it is true defilement (the children did not, in all likelihood, know that she was a zombie, but they had received the order not to establish any physical connection, and even less of an emotional one, with her). In contrast, Adeline D. does not forget to depict her own arms when she draws herself in the middle of this house.

Physically, Adeline D. presents obvious signs of bodily neglect. Her nails are long and dirty, and she seldom washes herself. Her symptoms combine amnesia, sporadic deliria (of the mystical variety, describing "invisible people" around her), frequent episodes of sexual hyperexcitation, problems with concentration, and temporospatial disorientation. She has had no other language difficulty outside of a few episodes of coprolalia. For Dr. Girard, her medical chart is completely superimposable onto that of other patients described in the vast biomedical literature dedicated to victims of the consumption of meat contaminated by tetrodotoxin, particularly in terms of her recurrent absences. A bit after his "rebirth," Clairvius Narcisse had episodes of aphasia and/or dysarthria that gradually became less and less frequent over time.

Of course, Adeline D. endured a comprehensive series of further examinations. Biologically speaking, a complete assessment was completed that did not reveal any anomaly (thyroid assessment—T3, T4, TSH—blood, urinary, toxicological). On April 24, 2014, she also had an MRI with an injection of a contrast agent (gadolinium) (this is perhaps the first time that a subject considered to be a zombie underwent this type of additional examination). This assessment shows:

> Progressive cortical changes without relationship to the age of the sick individual. Normal convolutions of the brain and of the cerebellum. Discreet widening and deepening of the cortical sulci with frontal and parietal predominance, symmetrical ventricular system of normal size. Basal ganglia, internal capsule, corpus callosum, and thalamus and region of the hippocampus are all normal. Sella turcica, pituitary gland, and parasellar structures are all normal. No pathology at the level of the cerebellopontine angle nor in the two hemispheres. Development and pneumaticity of the paranasal sinuses and of the mastoid part are all normal. Normal orbital canal.

Put another way, Adeline D. is the site of a frontoparietal atrophy of the cortex. It is the only anomaly shown with regard to the brain, which does not explain her condition at all. Could her behavior have more of a functional cause than a natural one?

An electroencephalogram (EEG) was also completed. Here are the results:

> At the beginning of the plot, during her sleep induced with chloral hydrate, we record a distribution of peaks with right frontal and parietal predominance, parietal-occipital, and left frontal-temporal. To the right, we also register brief flashes of activity toward the end of sleep, the amplitude of the route diminishes and we record slow waves and peaks. The hyperpnoea shows wide periodic flashes separated by

periods of decrease in amplitude creating the impression of spasms. At rest, we measure a wider activity in the right and left frontal-parietal and a dispersal of slow waves and peaks of weak amplitude on the other branches. Other stimulations are not applied. In total, it is route suggestive of multiple irritative sites. There is no sign of anoxic coma.

This examination thus shows that Adeline D. spends her time (if it can be put this way) having epileptic attacks, and her MRI shows that it has probably been happening for a long time because she is already showing frontoparietal atrophy. Her behavioral problems are thus the sum of frontal attacks and of the chronic psychosis of untreated epileptics. . . . It is impossible to determine whether it is the effects of a possible former massive dose of tetrodotoxin.

Outside of her sister who initially recognized her, her "children" come to see her from time to time (implicitly confirming her identity although, for her part, she does not recognize them), but never her husband, who lives near Cap-Haïtien. Adeline D. does not want too many visits and, above all, she does not handle well being an object of curiosity. When her children come accompanied by other individuals, she sometimes rejects them violently.

But she knows to be grateful towards those who came to her aid. One morning, on her school notebook from which she had torn out a page, she wrote (in Creole) to Dr. Girard:

> My dear NPA Director [National Penitentiary Administration], in truth, I will tell you how, now, I am content, Dr. Girard, for you have eased my mind and made me happy by having me come here to Port-au-Prince and by making me leave Limonade. If I must die, I thank God, full of faith. You did not leave me outside to beg. Thank you.

Dr. Girard is not afraid of her. He even brought her to his home one day when he was having a party. She danced there. She danced a lot, even. And with a lot of people who were unaware that she was a zombie. If they had known, the reactions would not necessarily have been violent. They would have sooner sparked a high level of curiosity. But in the hospital, my colleague does not desire any such behaviors. All personnel know exactly who Adeline D. is, what her history is, and accept her without batting an eye. Even the new student interns, when they arrive, are immediately brought into line: do not judge her, simply care for her.

What is her future? Adeline D. has returned to the psychiatric hospital, but she has no ID papers and no legal existence. Aided by Maître Jeanty, Dr. Girard is going to try to expand Haitian law and have the stolen life of this woman recognized (while hoping that this recognition will set a precedent for other present and future cases). One possible idea is to go to the registry and file a late declaration so that she can be rehabilitated into society. As she is used to her new name of Mirlande Antoine, that is how she will be called and legally recognized from now on (and not Adeline D.). It is thus not a question of a birth certificate (and even less a question of a "rebirth certificate"), but of a declaration of acknowledgement that will be certified by a court of law. As for her parentage, that is a difficult matter. . . . The exact name will probably be "of unknown parents," for lack of a better alternative, while further genetic evaluation is pending. Appended to this acknowledgement could be a certificate of adoption by the rest of the family, to reintegrate her into the group.

This is not Dr. Girard's first zombie. He had previously taken care of a woman who had reappeared in the town of Beaumont, had begun to speak, and had then suddenly disappeared after having been threatened.

Another of his zombie patients was Jeanne Jacqueline, a native of Gonaïves, declared dead at the mortuary on September 12, 2011, and found quite alive thirteen months later. She had hardly spoken at all since her zombification, continuously keeping her head lowered, her eyes half-closed, and appearing completely lifeless. She was filmed on several occasions. One can thus see her decked out in a red striped sweater that bears the image of Padre Pio, unintelligibly articulating a few mystical words: "I am Jesus. Jesus is with me," while refusing to be touched. Recognized by her own parents and also by the rest of her family, she died from cholera a few years afterwards.

Jeanne Jacqueline's case is truly unique because her parents wanted to go to the cemetery of Savane Bout near Saint-Raphaël (on the north side of the island) to bury her. Why this specific cemetery? In all Haitian cemeteries, the first dead person to be buried is regarded as Baron Samedi (they commonly call him simply "Baron"). Yet the first person interred at Savane Bout was a mute. One cannot, therefore, ritually exhume the dead in this place, because Baron's prior permission is necessary—and, in the present instance, he cannot give it, since it is impossible for him to express himself. This cemetery, hidden deep within the backcountry, an almost complete guarantee of *post mortem* peacefulness, is very trendy. Therefore, there are no zombies in this cemetery. Except that in this instance, the hearse never arrived! Along the way, the car had an accident, and the casket was thrown onto the roadside. A little while later, Jeanne Jacqueline returned home. . . .

CHAPTER 14

LOUBEAU FUNERAL HOME

Since 1962, the *Pax Villai* establishment has been tucked into the heart of a vast territory of gardens and lawns on the edge of the national highway leading to Toussaint Louverture International Airport in Port-au-Prince. Several single-story buildings are dedicated to the cold-room storage of corpses, to their embalming for international transport, and to the presentation of caskets intended for funeral ceremonies.

I interview an employee handling registrations and the stock of caskets. She tells me that now, nearly ten percent of deceased individuals undergo cremations (which represents two to three people per week), whereas there were around two to three cremations per month before the earthquake of 2010. This practice is constantly rising and, for some (beginning with Mr. Loubeau, the proprietor of the establishment), it is the best way to fight against the possible appearance of zombies. Even if it means incinerating individuals who are only in a state of apparent death, this would be an expeditious solution.

The wooden and metal caskets, mostly American imports (Batesville, Indiana), are all padded with foam cushions and are covered in spotless white polyester. The caskets have a bolt on the side. They open mid-length in order to display the top half of the body. Once locked inside, the subject cannot get out on his or her own due to the safety mechanism. In systematic fashion, all bodies receive an intra-abdominal and intrathoracic injection of disinfecting agents; if national or international transport is scheduled, then a complete embalming is carried out with an exsanguination followed by an intravascular and intravisceral injection of the formalin variety of preserving agents.

CHAPTER 15

MIREILLE THE *MAMBO*

It is through the intermediary Herlyne Blaise that I am able to get in touch with Mireille Aïn, a Haitian *mambo* of French origin. A former executive of cultural administration trained in the schools of the French Republic, one day she was "called" during a trip to Haiti and she decided to stay there. She only interrupts her stay for a few weeks every year in order to undergo medical treatment in Guadeloupe.

At first, everything went poorly for her because Vodou corresponds to a way of thinking that is completely different from the one in which she was raised. During her initial trances, she remembers being asked what was happening. "It was very perturbing," she admits. Afterwards, from trance to trance and from discussion to discussion, she noticed that the standards in which she was raised are not the only ones and that others are not necessarily bad. She was initiated in Max Beauvoir's peristyle in Mariani.

The relationship with nature seems to her much more interesting in Vodou since it is not an adoption of humanity's exploitation of the earth and of nature. "If you do not have leaves to care for, if you do not have nature with you, you are lost." It is within the everyday environment that you best notice the *loas* . . . which has enabled her to break away from her European roots completely. *Mambo* Mireille recognizes an absolute simplicity in the community of Vodou practitioners; "They have never said to me, 'You are white. Stay here. Do not enter.' On the contrary. They have initiated me into almost everything. Vodou is a sharing and a generosity that you do not find elsewhere."

In fact, Vodou is a very open religion: "No Vodou practitioner, no *houngan*, no *mambo* will refuse an initiation to anyone because he is Protestant, Catholic, homosexual, etc." It is a religion in which woman has her rightful place. It is a religion in which she is whole. The relationship with the body is completely different (unlike conduct at church which is very conventional, with a rather strict dress code and etiquette). In Vodou, there are dances, trances, etc., interpreted by colonists as licentious orgies. If the assistants drink, the initiates (*hounsis*) drink relatively little "at least at the beginning of the ceremony." *Mambo* Mireille has never seen unrest, but if unrest were to arise, particularly among the *guédés* equipped with sticks in the shape of a penis, it would not be very serious, since "it is death that fertilizes life." In touching them (or even striking them squarely) with their ritual objects, they fertilize them.

The last *déchoukaj* goes back at least thirty years. At the fall of the Duvalier regime on February 7, 1986, dozens of Tontons Macoutes and *houngans* were lynched or burned alive in the middle of the street, accused of acts of sorcery in support of the dictatorship. In the months that followed, Protestant preachers intensified this repression, which was accompanied by the vandalizing of multiple *hounfors*. Following these events, the *hounsi* joined together in a National Confederation of Haitian Vodou Practitioners, uniting sixteen Vodou organizations from the island. They launched special radio and television stations: Canal 11 in Jacmel, Radio Guinée, Chaîne Caraïbe, etc. They became involved in environmental conservation, as they consider the numerous springs, rivers, creeks, etc., to be sacred, and they participate in their decontamination or their clean-up in accordance with the full respect of the *loas*. When a tree is sacred, they say that it is *servi*. This means that they make sacrifices intended to honor the tree's presence and the *loa* who lives there.

This *mambo* has never encountered a zombie, but she has heard a lot of talk about the process of zombification. She often visits a few pastors who see zombies "because it's their job," but what is certain is that zombification exists. It is not an act of malfeasance. It is an act of social justice, a traditional way of providing justice. A person who disturbs an area, "and I mean really disturbs it (raping girls, making babies all over the place, stealing land, and provoking great disorder). . . . You know the country's judicial system? Justice follows its course . . . twenty years later, there isn't anyone left." Except that then there is one additional zombie. Thus, traditionally, one went to see the *houngan* or the *mambo* who did not perform zombification themselves. Once the problem was explained to them, they tried to solve it in the most peaceful way possible by going to meet or by summoning the different parties while attempting to find an arrangement using their moral authority; "But sometimes, when you wander too much, that isn't enough." Then, out of spite, one went next to meet with the Society head. That is why secret societies have very bad reputations.

Mambo Mireille is part of a Society (which usually includes thirty to forty individuals), so she knows very well how things function. In the event of a complaint, one meets with the accused person several times. One talks to him or her, but also questions the plaintiff, because some of them lodge a complaint for the pleasure of complaining or out of malice, with the goal of regaining land, etc. This *mambo* remembers having had a plaintiff sentenced to pay several thousand *gourdes* for a wrongful accusation and for "having unnecessarily disturbed the Society."

There are several types of punishment (money, *coup de poudre*, etc.) within the Societies, and zombification is truly the most significant. But when one decides to zombify an individual, one is choosing to condemn him to a loss of identity, possessions, everything. This is also done because Vodou does not allow the death penalty. Vodou does not kill—at least, it does not kill humans. Therefore, when someone is zombified, he is immersed in a type of coma, then removed from it a few hours later (so that the coma will be reversible, for if the individual stays too long in his casket, he will end up dying), taken out of the cemetery, and passed through what they call the "trails of enchantment." Then another Society takes charge of him and brings him to the other end of the republic. Zombies generally always end up far from home.

When one talks with *mambo* Mireille about zombies working in the sugar cane fields, she admits laughing about this widespread fantasy:

> They are guarded. When they say that it is for farming, you have to laugh a lot because given the price of labor in Haiti. . . . Zombies have to be taken care of. They have to be fed and monitored because they are not very autonomous. You have to ensure that they remain in good shape—perhaps not health wise, but at least that they remain alive. You have to make specific food for them. In short, it's a lot of constraint for a yield that is practically worthless. The zombie has automatic movements, in fact, but he performs them at an extremely slow pace.

At the time of the American occupation, many grabbed hold of the phenomenon of zombification. No effort was spared to demonize Vodou practitioners. Many individuals feigned cases of "demonic" possession while serving pastors and/or politicians. During this period, both false zombies and real zombies (in retaliation) experienced an extremely significant rise in frequency. "This is when you began to see cattle with golden teeth throughout the Republic." The expression hides a tradition. When one sent an individual to the other end of the country during a zombification and news comes back to the head of the Society that the zombie has arrived at his final destination spot, one then sacrifices a steer that is presented in front of the entire community to indicate that justice has been served.

A second meaning, just as mundane, also exists for this expression. When a *bokor* senses death approaching for one of the zombies over which he is keeping watch, he transforms him into a steer so that he might either be killed for butchering or die a natural death. But when chopping up the pieces or even when still inside the market stalls, one realizes "that the steer had golden teeth" (in other words, that it was no more and no less than a man magically transformed into an animal).

For *mambo* Mireille, if there is a common toxicological basis for *poudre zombi*, each Society, when it understands the mysteries of zombification, has its own specificities, sometimes using more *fufu* fish (some preferring the bones, others preferring the liver), sometimes more Datura, etc.

You have to understand once and for all that Vodou medicine—because it is part of medicine due to the fact that it concerns biological preparations—is composed of a physical part (with plants, animals, and minerals) and a spiritual or mystical part that cannot be exported.

In other words, when Wade Davis and his North American colleagues worked on samples of *poudre zombi*, they only scratched the surface of this phenomenon. The manufacturing process is extremely long. It sometimes takes several months to gather the ingredients; some plants are not easy to find, and it will thus be necessary to travel or send away for them. Then comes the period of mystical preparation, which can also be very long.

For *mambo* Mireille, there can be no zombie without the mystical preparation. Some people with a lot of money were able to buy *poudre zombi* and they gave some of it to a few victims who were immersed in a deep coma, but they never became zombies. "Zombification is based on an understanding conveyed by Vodou to the human personality, to the *ti-bon-anj* and the *gwo-bon-anj*, for example. It plays thereupon as well."

They always talk about a form of zombie that is spectacular, those that are half robot and that have lost their intellect. They only have vital functions left. But there is also what they call the *zombi bouteille*. When someone dies, at a funeral ceremony in a *lakou*, for example, one takes a bottle, wraps it in a sheet, and places it in the bottom of the vault. Then the casket is placed in front and the vault is closed with a wall of stone or cement. The goal is to lock everything so that this zombie will not be removed. Inside the bottle is a part of this person's soul which, after a particular ritual, can be used. In such cases, it is a zombie that is not visible. Often, when a *houngan* or a *mambo* dies, one pays close attention so that he or she is not exhumed. People stand vigil over him for the time that is required and do not bury him anywhere else. *Mambo* Mireille knows a *mambo* who had a false burial. Her casket was filled with stones and the real body was buried elsewhere in secret in order to not arouse the *bokors'* keen interest. "Clearly, I can tell you that she is not in her official grave in the cemetery."

In Brazil, in the *candomblé*, the same protection rituals are practiced. When a *fils-de-saint* (*filho-de-santo*) dies, they beat the drums in front of the body for seven days.[1] "You must not let him out of your sight."

The cemeteries in Haiti have several distinctive features. At the entrance, there is the grave of Baron (Samedi) that can be a false sepulcher or it might match the oldest sepulcher in the cemetery. Baron Lacroix corresponds to Baron Samedi, but within a *lakou*, because in Haiti, a person can be buried at home. If it is a woman, they will call her Grande Brigitte. Offerings will be made there since they are the guardians of the cemetery. The other characteristic of Haitian cemeteries is that they are open continuously (including at night).

Some individuals still talk about a practice that takes place less and less often, the *travail cimetière*. Others speak of *exorcismes* (although this word does not at all take on the same meaning as in Christian Europe): when an individual is very ill, they go to bury him in a hole dug in the actual cemetery or in the courtyard of the *lakou*. While singing a ritual, they stretch his body out on a banana leaf even before he has died. The goal is to awaken him from his illness and to rouse him so that he will fight against what is attacking him.

Another ritual that unfolds in Haitian cemeteries is the *manger pauvre*. When a *houngan* or a *mambo* opts for such a ceremony, he informs the cemetery caretaker and arrives with all of his *hounsi*. Coffee and food are placed on funerary stones, then served to all those who pass by. Afterwards, everyone leaves. It is an act of Vodou charity, but in this case, it is the living that they feed.

The crosses at the entrances of cemeteries are frequently the object of rituals and sacrifices. On the cross in Jacmel, for example, dozens of melted candles still stick to the stone, but also feathers and the blood of chickens. As *mambo* Mireille says mischievously, "There is no worse fate than being a hen in Haiti." The Vodou practitioner can go there alone or he can be accompanied by *houngans* or a *mambo*. Each offering is connected to a request made by the intermediary of the ancestors or of the *loas*: healing, or a wish, but also a desire for justice. If Baron Samedi is not associated with justice, his spouse, on the other hand, is linked to it.

In Haiti, as outside of the country, Vodou is under-recognized. With the concordat, the campaigns of *rejeté, le déchoucaj,* etc., Vodou has not had (and still does not have) more than a few friends. This poor image is skillfully maintained by Protestant congregations. According to *mambo* Mireille, nearly eight percent of children are in congregational schools, where they begin to teach them very early that "Vodou is the devil." Each year, between Christmas and New Year's Day, one or more priests shriek while declaring, with great movement of the chasuble, that Vodou practitioners kill children during "black masses" and grind them in large mortars to make magic potions of them.

There are two development models in Haiti that coexist, but which are not yet in dialogue with each other: the Westernized model, on the one hand, and the popular mainstream model, founded on acceptance, exchange, and justice rendered by the Societies, on the other. Each one tries to destroy the other, but the forces are not equal, because money is not on the side of the Vodou practitioner. After the earthquake, funds were largely freed up for rebuilding cathedrals, churches, seminaries, and parochial schools, but almost no funding was acquired to repair peristyles. No Vodou schools exist. This does not prevent a number of Christians from performing Vodou worship services at the same time.

CHAPTER 16

NATIONAL BUREAU OF ETHNOLOGY

In a nook of the National Bureau of Ethnology near the ruins of the Presidential Palace in Port-au-Prince, half-hidden by bookcases filled with assorted books, a *makaya* Vodou altar is kept, containing numerous characters with human skulls. These figurines have a frightening appearance, with bodies made of papier-mâché, patched clothing, doll heads that look like those of children, and animal horns, with everything painted in bright red, purple, or black. The set is covered with a substantial layer of grey dust and carbon black. One can make out a baby with three horns (it is a used doll); a red statue; a bottle to which are attached two legs, a hand, and a mini liquor bottle on its head with a frightening face; an individual with two female heads carrying a baby in its arms; a small fire pit with two bottles positioned one on top of the other; a person on a chair whom another person is in the process of strangling; and yet another rather frightening individual with human hair that falls onto a skeletonized face, carrying in its right hand a bottle and in its left a tiny baby. It includes *bizango* dolls (corresponding to the indigenous army, the secret face of Vodou—in other words, secret societies) originating from several altars of ancestors located in the northern part of the island. Where did the skulls come from? Either from salvage operation in cemeteries, or from important initiates who wished to give this part of their bodies and their souls after death as a gift to be used in the ritual.

The Musée du quai Branly (Paris) recently acquired such a *bizango*. Around one meter in height, it features a human face that is shrouded with a dark taffeta, covered with mirror shards, mounted on a body made of red fabric, holding a pair of intentionally bent scissors in its right hand and a walking stick in its left hand. X-rays now allow us to understand better "the anatomy of masterpieces" (to use Christophe Moulherat's expression): in fact, it has been possible to confirm the (previously suspected) presence of a real human skull inside this Vodou fetish. Anthropologically speaking, it is the skull of an adult subject of feminine morphology. Its appearance accords with a Black Caribbean origin. Is it the remains of a former *mambo* belonging to this secret society? The skull is completely skeletonized, and almost no organic remains are left (neither brain, muscle, nor skin). Shards of glass (mirror) have been affixed to the eyes, ears, nose, and mouth, consistent with the other shards on the rest of the body. Hardly a single tooth is in position; many fell out before death (molars). Others fell out after death (decomposition, putrefaction, moving of the skull) and only a few root fragments remain. The examination of the rest of the subject does not reveal any other skeletal remains.

CHAPTER 17

OTHER ZOMBIES . . . DEAD OR ALIVE

The Vodou religion acknowledges the existence of three different zombie types (which, in reality, are interrelated): the astral zombie relates to an element of the soul that can be transmuted according to the will of the person who possesses it (usually the *bokor*); the corpse zombie is a "living dead" that can be forced to work; the marsh zombie corresponds to a former zombie of the flesh who has returned to a state of living.

These different types of "false dead" are literally part of the cultural and religious heritage of Haiti. It is also reported—and over time these anecdotes have become real fairytales and legends—that in 1918, the factory of the Haitian-American Sugar Corporation (Hasco) in Port-au-Prince needed cheap manual labor and that a foreman (Ti Joseph) and his wife (Croyance) had come accompanied by nine confused men dressed in rags with a glassy look and their feet dragging. These men were presented as peasants originating from the mountains at the border with the Dominican Republic, real bumpkins, but who were gifted with tremendous strength. Hired in spite of everything, they accomplished an incredible amount of work from sunup to sundown. When evening came, they ate only unsalted millet porridge. They were obviously zombies . . . and Vodou tradition reports that if a zombie one day eats salt or meat, then he becomes aware of his horrible condition, cries all the tears from his body, and immediately returns to the path that leads toward his grave (in other words, his natural place). That is exactly what happened. One morning when Ti Joseph was away, Croyance decided to "give them a smile" after having led them to a religious procession (without arousing the slightest response in them). She gave some peanuts to each of them, but they were salty! What was supposed to happen happened. The zombies began to bay for blood and, yelling, they fled all the way back to their native village (Morne-au-Diable).

> These dead walking in single file were seen by the villagers . . . on the market square. The crowd approached and each one recognized a father, a brother, a wife, or a daughter that had been buried several months earlier. The majority understood immediately that they had been snatched from their graves and that they were zombies, but a few of them hoped that a miracle had taken place on this Easter day and that they had been resurrected. They ran up to embrace them. But the zombies crossed the square at their sleepwalker pace without recognizing anyone, and as they were moving along the pathway toward the cemetery, a woman whose daughter was walking with the dead flung herself in front of her shouting, and she begged her to stay. But the girl placed her icy feet on her and all of the others walked on the poor woman without seeing her.[1]

Without hesitation, they headed for the cemetery and, each one finding his or her own grave, they began to scratch the ground then lay down in their sepulchers. Immediately, they began to rot. They say, indeed, that while making zombies, *bokors* have the power to prevent their decomposition.

The peasants' vengeance was not long in coming, and a spell was fashioned against the *bokor*.

> They took up a collection in the village and with the money and Ti Joseph's shirt [stolen during the night by an accomplice], the men went to the home of another *bokor* living in Trou Caïman who made a death *ouanga* in a dark sack, pierced it with needles, rubbed it with goat excrement, and wrapped it in rooster feathers soaked in blood. Furthermore, in the event that the *ouanga*, weakened by Ti Joseph's counter

magic, would not be fast enough, they sent a few strong men into the lowlands who waited for Joseph, and one evening they cut off his head with machetes.

This anecdote is told by a certain William Seabrook who heard it from a Haitian farmer (Constant Polynice). In the 1920s, Seabrook had the chance to observe three zombies closely, cutting cane in a field near Picmy, each with a machete in his hand and under the supervision of a young woman (their caretaker):

> My first impression of the three zombies, who were continuing to work, was that they had something truly bizarre; they had automatic movements. I couldn't see their faces, hung as they were towards the ground. But Polynice took one by the shoulder and gestured to him to stand up straight. Docile as an animal, the man got back up and what I saw then gave me a painful shock. The most horrible thing was the gaze, or rather the absence of one. His eyes were dead, as if blind, and devoid of expression. His entire face was thus, expressionless, incapable of expression.[2]

Seabrook does not stand by at this simple sight, but takes hold of one of this creature's hands, which he finds limp, hard, human, and calloused.

We can agree that the Hasco zombies story, with their putrefaction upon returning to the original grave, more or less resembles an old wives' tale, and, with the time that has passed, it is very difficult to extract a grain of truth from it. Nevertheless, attracted by this concept of "living dead," scientists have been looking, since the American occupation, to untangle what is true from what is false: they meet supposed zombies, examine them medically, conduct tests, and capture the data. Thus, in 1937, the African-American ethnologist Zora Neale Hurston earns a Guggenheim fellowship to go to Haiti and Jamaica in order to conduct research on the local culture. She succeeds in entering secret societies and in attending numerous Vodou rituals. With Seabrook, also initiated into Haitian Vodou, Hurston thus became one of the first non-Haitian witnesses to describe an encounter with a zombie. In fact, Hurston's investigation not only constitutes one of the oldest anthropological accounts on the subject, but the American ethnologist was also the author of the first photographic snapshot of a zombie.

Hurston reports that in October or November 1936, a woman who was wandering dazed and naked was apprehended in the valley of Artibonite. She was heading towards a farm where her brother worked as a foreman, and it was while the workers were scaring her off that her brother recognized the sister he had buried twenty-nine years earlier. She was said to have been named Felicia Felix-Mentor, and she had died in 1907 following a sudden coma. The family was convinced that the deceased woman had been a victim of poisoning. Hurston came to see her at the Gonaïves hospital:

> We found the zombie in the courtyard of the hospital. They had just placed her dinner in front of her, but she was not eating. At the moment that she sensed our arrival, she broke the branch of a shrub and began to use it to clean the dust from the ground and the table on which her food sat. Her two doctors were saying kind things to her and were trying to reassure her, but she seemed to hear nothing. One of the doctors then uncovered her head for a moment (she had covered it with a cloth), but she quickly knocked his arms and hands up over her as if she were attempting to move aside things that she feared. Finally, the doctor forced her to remain with her head uncovered and . . . the sight became horrible. Her face was expressionless, with dead eyes. Her eyelids were white like they had been burned by acid.[3]

The affair attracted international attention and sparked a fierce debate within the scientific community. Haitian psychiatrist Louis P. Mars attempted to demystify this case by means of an X-ray of the woman's ankle. He noted that Felix-Mentor had suffered a fracture of the ankle, whereas the presumed zombie had not.

Zora Hurston also described another zombie: Marie, a young girl who died in 1909. Five years after her death, former classmates noticed her at the window of a house in Port-au-Prince. The story causes a good deal of commotion and the community is troubled by this sudden reappearance. To definitively end the debate, they have the casket opened, and in it they discover a skeleton that is too long for the container and does not match

Marie's height. The clothing that the "deceased" was wearing during her inhumation was carefully folded next to the bones. It was rumored that Marie had been dug up and used as a zombie until the *bokor* who had made her died. The widow of the Vodou sorcerer then returned her to a Catholic priest, who sent her out of Haiti in deepest secrecy. She was then placed in a convent where her brother visited her several years later.

How can we know what the truth is? For Zora Hurston, zombification was the punishment for those who had betrayed the mysteries of the secret Haitian societies. But no one believed her. "Zora Hurston is very superstitious," the French ethnologist Alfred Métraux condescendingly wrote.

"The army of darkness" is the name given to a very special faction of the Tontons Macoutes, in the stranglehold of the Duvaliers, between 1958 and 1986. In Haiti, the fear of sorcerers capable of making zombies is so great that that it keeps all fantasies alive to the point where it has a social and even a political impact. The prestige of secret societies is indeed increased by the mystery surrounding their power associated with Vodou practices. If secret societies had a crucial role to play at the time of the revolt against French colonial domination that gave Haiti its independence, these societies continued long afterwards to influence the history of the Republic, and were used by Haitian leaders such as François Duvalier as elements of their political power. Until the overthrow of the Duvalier regime in 1986, the rumor was maintained that their secret police, the Tontons Macoutes (from the name of the folkloric villain who steals and eats children), included in its ranks numerous zombies enslaved by secret Vodou potions, but also that the dictator himself was filled with incredible magical powers.

In 1966, the English anthropologist Francis Huxley reported that a Catholic priest confided in him that he had seen a zombie in the process of gnawing on the rope that bound his wrists, then drinking salty water (which symbolically awakens the dead). Shortly afterwards, he was able to say his name. They found his family; they located his aunt, who confirmed the identity of this man, and explained that he had been buried four years earlier.

At 1:15 p.m. on May 2, 1962, the now-famous Clairvius Narcisse, *alias*

Louis Ozias, passes away at Albert-Schweitzer Hospital in the city of Deschapelles, a short distance from his *lakou* in Estère. He had been admitted three days earlier with a fever and sore muscles, spitting blood, before quickly sinking into a coma. His death was certified by two Western physicians and the cause of death was recorded in the medical record as "malignant hypertension and uremia." The body, identified by his family, was buried the next day. Eighteen years later, a man claiming to be Clairvius Narcisse gets in touch with one of his sisters (Angelina), confirming that he had been bewitched and zombified. He describes his state from that point as conscious, but, paralyzed at the moment of his death and burial, he was powerless to defend himself against his exhumation by a group of men presumed to be the *bokor* and his gang. For two years, he was beaten and enslaved on a plantation until another worker killed his abductor (or, according to another version, until one of his guards forgot to give him his daily dose of drugs). Clairvius then got away in a state that he describes as dreamlike and completely sluggish, without any of his own will any more. Having finally regained complete consciousness, he chose to remain out of sight until the death of the brother with whom he was on bad terms before his zombification, and whom he had accused of having paid the *bokor* to poison him. Holding his Bible in one hand, he ended up dying many years later, in all likelihood of natural causes (pneumonia). His family buried him in Haiti in a cemetery belonging to an American mission (he had become an evangelist).[4] Clairvius Narcisse did not, however, have one of the characteristic signs of zombies (and of *guédés*, those *loas* of the dead): a twangy voice.

It was Lamarque Douyon, a psychiatrist of Haitian origin working at McGill University in Montreal, who seized upon the case of this patient, then specialized in the scientific and practical study of the phenomena of zombies, but also in specific treatment before they were brought to the point of reappearance and reintegration into the civilian world. Douyon, accompanied by ethnobotanist Wade Davis, also worked on the case of Natagete Joseph. Around sixty years of age, she had been "killed" in 1966 during a financial disagreement, then recognized in 1979 wandering around in her native village by the police officer who, in the absence of a doctor, had pronounced her dead.

Another zombie case appeared in 1979 when a young thirty-year-old woman named Francina Ileus was discovered in a catatonic state by a friend. Francina was buried in the family tomb located next to her house on February 23, 1976, the same day that she died as a result of a brief feverish illness. Two distinctive features made this woman especially believable. Firstly, Francina was recognized by her mother, who confirmed her presumed identity thanks to a mark on her face (a childhood scar present on her temple). Her seven-year-old daughter, her brothers and sisters, the local priest, as well as other villagers recognized her. Next, when the grave was opened on instructions from a local tribunal, the casket was thoroughly examined. It was filled with rocks, but there was no body. Having become Douyon's patient at the psychiatric hospital in Port-au-Prince, the one they nicknamed *Ti Femme* remained mute and incapable of feeding herself for years. She was labeled "mentally handicapped" or as having "catatonic schizophrenia." She had apparently been zombified for having refused to marry the man that her family had chosen for her (while she carried in her belly a child belonging to another man)[5] or, according to other versions, by her jealous husband after she had had an affair.

Upon clinical examination, she looked a lot younger and thinner than in a family photo take a few years earlier. She continually kept her head in a lowered position and walked very slowly, all stiff, hardly managing to move her arms. In terms of her muscles, the presence of a decrease in tone was noted, but there was no abnormal flexibility. She did not answer any questions, but occasionally murmured a few incomprehensible and banal words. She remained completely insensitive to events. The electroencephalogram (EEG) taken in the psychiatric hospital was normal. During all the years in which she received these treatments, Ti Femme never cooperated with the slightest psychological evaluation nor with useless attempts at social reinsertion. The neuroleptics had no effect on her symptoms. While she was at a market during hospital leave, she was immediately recognized by the crowd as being a zombie.

At the Psychiatric Center of Port-au-Prince, near the end of his life, Dr. Douyon also took on the care of two additional individuals considered to be zombies: Medula Charles, the only daughter of a family from Gros-Morne, twenty-four years of age, and Wilfried Pierre, a young man thirty years of age, a native of Dessource. Both were extremely emaciated and malnourished when they were hospitalized. They experienced significant problems with concentration and were victims of frequent hallucinations. Even though they were both able to recognize their parents, they spoke of the *bokors* as their *papas* who had held them in custody. These two zombies had been found in the valley of Artibonite, but they had nothing to do with each other. The first had been zombified for a questionable matter pertaining to the denunciation of a thief, and had even become pregnant as a zombie. We know nothing of what became of the child. Neither of the families accepted that zombies had returned to live among them.

In 1973, Jean Kerboull, missionary at the seminary of Saint-Jacques (Port-au-Prince) in the Haitian countryside, delivered two accounts of zombies. The first was named Exilus, a native of the region of Cayes. He "died" a short while after having insulted a *houngan*, and as a magical act never occurs in isolation in Haiti, at this exact moment, an old clock in the home of the deceased that no longer functioned suddenly began to work again. Two years afterwards, a certain Bossuet informed Exilus's father that his son was still alive and working in a house "as a slave." Meanwhile, his widow had remarried, but a sort of curse seemed to weigh on this new couple. The evening of the marriage ceremony, the groom fell from the bed several times, then he became completely helpless and seriously ill. He ended up leaving his new wife: "For the people, no doubt, this marital misfortune came from the fact that Exilus was still alive. The influence of the first husband, his zombie state, was paralyzing the poor man."[6]

The second account concerns a woman zombie, Médélia, whose identity was confirmed by a burn mark on her leg caused by a lighted candle that fell during her wake. She recounts the story herself after having recovered the entirety of her intellectual functions:

I was thirteen years old and I was a student of the sisters of the market town of Grande-Rivière when, one Sunday, I felt feverish while at the home of my aunt, Dorceline Dorcin (it's with her that my relatives from Milot had left me). She was a shopkeeper living close to the market. . . . During the night between Sunday and Monday, a strong ailment completely paralyzed me. In the morning, in everyone's opinion,

I was dead. Apparently, I was no more than a corpse; but I maintained enough lucidity to realize what was happening around me. Thus, I was aware of my transport from Grande-Rivière to Milot and conscious that my funeral was being conducted—the curate being away—by the sacristan. I was unable to follow the ceremonies; I had the impression of being in a hole that was completely black. Once in the pit, I heard the earth falling on my casket. And then, after a brief moment, I distinctly sensed a voice crying out: 'Soul . . . earth!' And quickly, I found myself outside, standing between two young people, still conscious, but without will. I was the object of my abductors and I remained the creature, and I remained the creature, of my abductors—until the day that, fearing the campaign of the Rejetés, they chased me and seven others away from them. After having left the cemetery, my two companions placed me in the hands of a gentleman who lived in a large house. . . . My main function, when they weren't sending me out to run errands, consisted of keeping the courtyard very clean, by means of constant sweeping and hoeing, and also by means of forbidding even the smallest animal to stay there, whether they were hens, pigs, or goats. Many times, my mission outside was to steal.[7]

Her *bokor* had changed her first name to Lina.

In February 1988, Wilfred Doricent, an adolescent from the village of Roche-à-Bateau (in the south of Haiti) quickly "succumbs" to a paralyzing illness. His family buries him without delay, but in September 1989, a friend recognizes him wandering in a neighboring village. The individual bore scars matching those of Wilfred. He was taciturn and mentally handicapped. Medical tests showed that he had suffered from cerebral lesions compatible with those caused by hypoxia. Belavoix Doricent, an uncle who had a local reputation as a *bokor* and with whom Wilfred's parents had a family quarrel, had been accused of having poisoned the teenager. In March 1990, this same Belavoix, prosecuted in court, was found guilty and sentenced to life imprisonment for poisoning. It is the only sentence that has ever been handed down for zombification.

In the first decade of the 21st century, seventeen zombies were found in miserable conditions near Jacmel (in the southern part of the island).

The identity of two of them, Joceline Relufe and Elitan Danroufer, dead and buried for several years, were confirmed by police authorities. The *bokor* responsible for their zombification was arrested in 2007. Shortly afterwards, in 2008, a *bokor* from Port-Margot (Ti Boss) had left nearly one thousand zombies for dead (this number is likely inflated by popular rumor . . .), one of which included a certain Ciliane who had been zombified three years prior. Upon the disappearance of her new master, as the children did not want to take over their father's activities, she returned to her family in Bande-du-Nord (near Cap-Haïtien). There, recognized by her family, she found her two children, her mother, and her husband.

In 2010, the Haitian police led an inquiry into the case of Adelin Seide, a young *houngan* of thirty years of age and a native of Fort-Liberté (Haïti). Seide had gone to a local tavern where he had shared some drinks with numerous guests, including a few strangers. He left with severe abdominal pains. After having suffered all night long, and despite the treatments given to him, the young man "died" the next morning (May 2, 2010) on the way to the hospital. Under Haitian law, the death was legally pronounced by two witnesses (who were not doctors), and a death certificate was duly signed. Seide's body was released from the charge of his brother, also a *houngan,* and was sent to a private morgue in Cap-Haïtien. The funeral ceremony took place in the Catholic church of Terrier-Rouge. Seide was buried on Wednesday, May 5, three days after his death. At 3:00 a.m. on May 6, the residents adjacent to the cemetery were awakened by a surprising racket. The police arrived and found the father of the deceased, Jeantery Seide, also a *houngan,* in front of his son's grave, a machete and a bottle in his hands. He maintained that he was coming to save his son from the "breeders of the dead." At the time of their subsequent inquiry, Haitian police found an empty casket and the young man alive. No complaint or legal charge was ever filed regarding this matter.

The belief in zombies exists in certain parts of Africa. The word zombie originates, incidentally, from the diverse ethnicities of Central Africa and directly relates to wandering spirits or ghosts.[8] In 1993, Sipho Mdletshe, a young man twenty-four years of age, was pronounced dead following a traffic accident in South Africa. His body was transported to the morgue and placed in a metal box. Two days later, Mdletshe, who was only in a coma, regained consciousness and began to call for help. Immediately rescued, he returned to his home to find his family, but he was eventually rejected by his fiancée who believed that he was a zombie returned to haunt her. . . .

Serious studies on zombie cases are rare. Some rather facetious North American university professors have used this word as a figure of speech to study, at the neurological level, changes related to states of low consciousness or brain death.[9] In 1997, the publication in *Lancet*—a medical journal with a worldwide reputation—of an article focusing on three cases of zombies medically examined by an English psychiatrist and his Haitian counterpart (Chavannes Douyon) was a bombshell within the scientific community.[10] After field investigations, clinical and supplementary examinations (scanning and genetic comparison with other members of the family, for example), practitioners were able to close the three selected files with various diagnoses: catatonic schizophrenia (for patient "FI," corresponding in all likelihood to Francina Ileus, seen above), post-anoxic brain damage with epileptic aftereffects, and loss of identity.

CHAPTER 18

VÉVÉ DRAWINGS

Night has long since fallen when I return to the home of Erol Josué. The car has difficulty weaving in and out through the labyrinth of tiny streets congested with fruit and pastry merchants. Children are running in the light of the headlights. It is warm outside. One sees stars above houses that are illuminated by pale light bulbs.

Before drawing a *vévé*, Erol the *houngan* went into the chamber of secrets to ask for permission to take cultural objects. Accompanied by the tracer, he must salute the four façades (the four cardinal points, or the forces of space). The individual who creates the drawing wears a black scarf, a *guédé* symbol, the ritual of the dead, and this *vévé* is called "cemetery" because it is dedicated to Baron Samedi, whose colors are black and purple. After drawing the *vévé*, the *houngan* also brings back several bottles from the chamber of secrets, corresponding to the drinks of Papa Guédé, which will be poured on the ground by way of a salute, necessary for the consecration of the space.

While awaiting the ceremony, I sit down on a bench. Everything takes its time in Haiti. In other words, everything ends up happening, but one never knows exactly when. Dogs bay for blood outside. The light from the candles jumps. The wind blows. The storm is not far away. In order to urge me to wait, Erol places a small red book in my hands with a *vévé* on the cover. It is the *vévé* of Erzulie Dantor. The book is a collection of Haitian

Vodou songs composed by Max Beauvoir. Under candlelight, I turn the pages, knowing neither in which country nor in which century I am. I read:

> The religion of the dead fully bridges the Vodou practitioner's belief in the immortality of the soul and in the freedom of will. . . . The rite of the dead and the appropriate rituals are, in reality, the achievement of the mystical works of each individual with regard not only to the vanished person, but even to the family, society, the community, and indeed even the State. This is why both friends and enemies of the deceased always participate. These rites bear witness to the belief that the individual's soul, composed of spiritual abundance . . . itself being unable to die, would have only temporarily lost its coherence. In a way, the spiritual fractions of the human being have just exploded and even separated themselves from the body. The life force of the deceased has just splintered into tiny spiritual particles that relate to being, intelligence, knowledge, will, consciousness, intuition, etc. This is why the said ceremonies of the *dessouni* are carried out for them, which are done sometimes even before or a bit after the physical death of the individual, the life force (*ti-bonanj*) leaving the body a long time before death. But the life force will have to return nearby the corpse or inside it, particularly at this social and critical moment for the individual or for society that we call *veillée* [vigil]. It will come back to reside in the funeral home and will sometimes remain there throughout the entire period of mourning. Then, the deceased individual comes to relive with the living the most memorable moments of his life, which are generally told by friends during these get-togethers. Sometimes, the deceased person even awakens during this time and expresses his final recommendations before departing once and for all.[1]

This reading reminds me of the anecdote that Laënnec Hurbon told a few days ago. Often during the wake or while the corpse is being prepared, loved ones or those who bathe the corpse talk with the deceased individual as if he were still alive, sometimes establishing real conversations (although, in all likelihood, a witness would only hear a single voice). The deceased, thus full of messages and recommendations, can comfortably depart for the invisible world.

> The most noteworthy parts of this rite of the dead are made up of chants, dances, and tales of a kind that are recounted there . . . and by the departure of this life force that can be awakened through a special ceremony called a *renvoie* that is most often performed forty-one days after this great departure. Let us mention that previously the use of *roucou* or *woucou* ("Rouge of the dead") to powder corpses also manifested similar thoughts, that of wanting to settle at all costs the unstable status of the deceased who failed to square his life's accounts, who, in a manner of speaking, stepped out of his duties (*defunctus* or deceased), and who wanders in uncertainty while awaiting his great departure.[2]

In a corner stands Louise Carmel-Bijoux, one of Erol's anthropology colleagues at the National Bureau of Ethnology. Quite petite, she melts into the shadows of the peristyle. She also examines the *hounsi* who is drawing the *vévé*. Three pigments are used for this drawing on the ground: a white corn powder, a red one made of crushed terra cotta (bricks), and a black one made of crushed charcoal. Louise explains to me that this art and this tradition are inherited from the Taíno, and they were taken up by slaves while perpetuating the tradition of the symbolic paintings of their divinities. For some people, it is the Taíno who left these images to black African slaves, who incorporated them into their rituals. She speaks in a low voice because it is a sacred moment. Well, to some extent. After ten minutes, no longer able to stand it, Erol goes up into his apartment and immediately comes back down with three very cold beers.

Once drawn, these images are used for the ceremony unfolding around them. These images say to the spirits, "We are ready. Come!" They attract the spirit's energy and serve to gather its approval for the ceremony. By means of this image, initiates and guests alike turn around and benefit from the drawings and the blessings of the *loas*. Once the ceremony is finished, this space, formerly considered sacred, no longer holds great significance, and the *vévé* can be erased (when it is not the dance itself that contributes to erasing it as the ceremony progresses).

Drawing a *vévé* is already a part of the ritual and of the ceremony (because the spirit is there). This drawing is usually done by candlelight, for it constitutes a preliminary step toward the light. For the pious person, the way that he dresses and the order of drawings made are not left to chance. Everything is weighed, felt, and reflected upon. The individual who draws must be "prepared," and his greeting to the *potomitan* already puts him in good standing.

The *vévé* of Baron Samedi features a cross sitting on top of a casket that adjoins a skeleton dressed in a top hat and cane, holding a bottle of alcohol. Two candles are then placed at the foot of the sketched cross and at the level of the genitals. Finally, Erol places seven bottles of alcohol among the different parts of the *vévé*. Thus built, it is fully consecrated to the god of the dead and of cemeteries, but also to those who accompany it, beginning with the life-*guédés*.

CHAPTER 19

IN THE CHAMBER OF SECRETS . . .

The *vévé* of Baron Samedi is now consecrated and the followers who danced, sang, and drank (a little) slowly disperse. While the silence and calm return, I resume my conversation with Erol Josué. He would like to convince me of the legitimacy of this Vodou justice that zombification represents: "To be made a zombie isn't random." It is a vengeance that is worse than prison or death, for the individual is deprived of all will and transformed into a real slave until his actual death. Only a few behaviors are particularly rebuked and lead to zombification: excessive ambition, fighting over inheritance, taking a woman from another man, and defamation. "Legal" errors are infrequent, if not almost unknown, or the object of totally unreasonable isolated acts committed by *bokors* who end up being zombified themselves by secret societies shortly thereafter.

In the Haitian future, the zombie will have to deal with the modernization of health systems enabling the detection of continuity of life before burial, but also his or her legal and social restoration once he or she emerges from the *bokor*'s clutches. At least, that is what hospital physicians and criminal lawyers have been ardently working on, hand-in-hand with educated *houngans* wishing to un-demonize Vodou and to allow its survival in the face of permanent pressure from Protestant churches—so that it is not Vodou that becomes a zombie.

Erol knows that a plane will take me back to France tomorrow. It is almost midnight. He is extremely tired. In spite of everything, before accompanying me to my car, he takes me by the arm and pulls me toward the back of the peristyle, towards the door of the chamber of secrets. "As the son of Zakpata, you have earned the right to see the other side of the mirror. . . ." Well-informed, Erol knows that I had, indeed, been initiated into Vodou near Abomey (Benin) on the blessing of Zakpata, protective god of the earth and of skin illnesses (mainly measles and smallpox).

He ritually knocks at the door to inform his *loas* that an initiate is requesting to enter. The wooden door creaks on its hinges. A few steps and I enter the first room, completely painted in blue pastel, by the light of a single candle that Erol is holding in his hand. All of Benin is there. First, I see the *loas blancs*, or *loas rada* (that come from the former Arada in present-day Benin), spirits mixed with Christian syncretism, in the center of which one can make out Damballa and his two garter snakes, Erzulie Fréda, and the Archangel Saint Michel. On the ground are the *marassa*, luck objects for deceased twins who have become spirits. Since they are children, they are on the ground near the earth which gave rise to them and which took them back. Nearby are the *makout zaka*, the working spirits consecrated to the farmers who are in the fields, represented by wicker saddlebags nailed to the walls (it is these spirits that bring knowledge of agriculture, and to which, in the month of May, one brings a quantity of food placed in said saddlebag). They adjoin peasant hats that are also hung on the wall. Large quantities of offerings are placed everywhere, including beverages and talismans.

This blue room connects to another one that is just as cramped. It is the red room (or the chamber of Erzulie Dantor), that of the *loas petro* (from the Creole world) and *congo* (from Central Africa). There are knives there (one of Erzulie's attributes, fittingly, presented as very austere, which breeds trust, but which, at the same time, defends itself and creates a distance), decorated bottles, twin luck objects, etc. In a corner, a small black casket (Erol advises me to not touch it), dried skulls (human and goat), cornbread, pairs of glasses, drinks that have been tampered with, a doll, a broom (used during therapeutic rituals to "sweep away evil"), a large cross painted red (more of a symbol of a crossroads or an intersection than Christian, in all likelihood), and a cologne that "brings luck." Between two altars, there is a basin filled with a depth of water that is used for treatments and ritual baths. Looking more closely, I see a small turtle at the bottom that is wading in slow motion. A personification of a divinity, she protects the *péristyle* (particularly from storms, in the same way as a lightning rod) and brings something deeper into the water (as if she were blessing the liquid by her presence). Nearby, on and under the altar tables, *pots de tête* are piled up. These are cups, glasses, or ceramics left by each initiate as a receptacle for their spirit. They contain several locks of hair or nail trimmings, and are closed by firmly tied fabric, and sometimes even with Scotch tape (so that the contents do not fly away). I look at Erol: "These locked-up souls thus exist. . . ." He gives a knowing smile.

The second door begins to creak. I must leave. I will come back.

POSTFACE

In Douala, at the beginning of 2003, an extraordinary case rallied crowds and the national press. A young man dead in a car accident had reappeared, wandering around the city like mentally ill individuals often do in Cameroon, and now he was speaking in English. Recognized by a relative, he was brought back to the family home where a growing, and soon paying, audience came to gather. There was much talk of reopening his grave to shed light on the mystery when a family from the Anglophone district recognized in press photos a son who had left town. The family had not received any news about him. A regrettable quarrel swelled up between the two parties, and if the real relatives ended up getting back their sick family member, some challenged their rights and persisted in thinking that the accident victim had certainly returned.[1] It is true that in the region, the business of "airplanes" that make nighttime round-trips between Cameroon and Europe or take slaves to work for their master on Mount Koupé one hundred kilometers from Mount Cameroon[2] are barely questioned. This is especially so since throughout Central Africa, it happens that if old graves dug along the roadside and threatened by public works must be raised, the grave will be empty or only contain bits and pieces of clothing. The skeleton, eaten away by the acidity of the laterite ground, has completely disappeared, which is considered proof that the dead individual has escaped. But if stories of ghosts and the living dead abound every-where, one may recall that France had to face some real zombies in the miserable soldiers of 1914–1918, traumatized and amnesiac, whose identity had been lost. Families, torn apart by the disappearance of a loved one, would fight with each other over the same sick person, all convinced that they recognized him, such as in the famous Anthelme Mangin case, the "unknown living soldier"[3] who inspired Giraudoux in *Siegfried et le Limousin* and Anouilh in *Le Voyageur sans bagage*. There, such as in Douala or in the Haitian cases recorded here (especially the case of Adeline D. or of Felicia), it is easily seen that confusion is maintained through questions of physical resemblance and the context of the affective disorder.

The literary figure of the zombie appears for the first time in what has been called the first French colonial novel written by the amazing adven-turer and "favorite of beauties," Pierre-Corneille Blessebois, who wanted "to serve Mars, Venus, and the Muses at the same time."[4] *Le Zombi du grand Pérou, ou La Comtesse de Cocagne* was published in 1697, in all likeli-hood in Rouen, where our hero perhaps saw his Normandy again after having been sentenced to the galleys and sold as an indentured servant in Guadeloupe. The text, a bit licentious[5] and particularly exotic, goes on to fascinate writers from Charles Nodier to the Surrealists. However, in this short novel in which prose and verse interleave, the zombie is, quite sim-ply, said barefooted countess, who desires to deceive her lover by want-ing to make herself invisible, which the author, whom she believes has magical powers, persuades her she is (it is about Blessebois himself who puts on a performance). Even if there is a bit of Erzulie in the countess, it is there more in the Molièresque farce than in the ethnography. But it is a three-hundred-year-old farce that reminds us to what extent the Creole world is full of these supernatural creatures that are, among other things, *manman-dlo* and *mamy-wata* in Africa, a siren in Homer's work, the *chouval trwa patt* that incarnates the devil, the "flyer" or *soucounyan*, the *baclou* of Guyana, a little golem that works for his master, or even the *dorlis* of Martinique, an incubus that comes to rape women, a "husband of the night," such as "the stick man," glorified by Ernest Pépin[6] and whose memory still haunted the Côte-sous-le-Vent in Guadeloupe not so long ago. All of these entities require that one wear a "protection" that is generally hidden on the individual, and a particular vigilance in certain places that one will avoid traversing at night.

Haiti, or Ayiti, "the mountainous island" (its Amerindian name), is obviously not a piece of Africa fallen into the Caribbean Sea, and the majority of religious traditions, such as the language or the cuisine there, are an amalgam of complex influences in which the memory of the Taíno (the indigenous Arawaks) is extinguished neither within the tradition nor in the genetics of its people.[7] The colonial order, reasonably transgressive if we believe what Blessebois says about it, is not made only of white masters and black slaves; there is also the enterprising and growing class of mulattos and free people of color that must assert itself, as well as the numerous "Petits Blancs," hired workers nicknamed "Red Bottoms" or "Thirty-Six Months," corresponding to the length of their contract, whose condition is wretched.[8] It is in this permeable society that figures of Creole syncretism form, such as the carnival that they celebrated on the old continent one thousand years before Vaval. And Africa, which in the Antillean imagination is the one and only mythical land, that of the lwa (loas) of Guinea, is certainly an immense continent with numerous, distinguished cultures. If the rootedness of Vodou is found in the Gulf of Benin, the word zombie is, for its part, Bantu and thus much more southern.[9] But the success of a term that sounds so far away and its integration into the Western imagination will hang on during the American military occupation of Haiti throughout the interwar period, a period in which cinema is ripe to recover and push towards the Grand-Guignol that which is, at its origin, the universal figure of the dead person called to life through sorcery practices.

This American episode emphasizes that the former and very prosperous colony of Saint-Domingue was built on a long series of tragedies that begins, as in other areas, with the genocide of Amerindians and slavery, but where natural disasters common throughout the arc of the Antilles have been on a particular increase on account of the social context, and where massacres and repression have been incomparably more atrocious than on the neighboring islands. Such a breeding ground could only be conducive to magic and sorcery and never far from politics,[10] if one refers

to characters such as the legendary Makandal.[11] Many intelligent ethno-
logical works have been devoted to Vodou, one of the most classic being
that of Alfred Métraux.[12] The present study does not have such a great
ambition. With portraits dedicated to noteworthy individuals and loca-
tions, it evokes more the travel experience of a young Paul Morand who,
in 1927, leads Métraux towards the poet and militant Jacques Roumain. It
is this great intellectual, who disappeared too early, who, starting in 1941,
bestows upon Haiti a National Bureau of Ethnology, a place where many
anthropological research studies will be developed. But from the initial
voyage that Dr. Charlier recounts to us emerges one tangible element in
the middle of this supernatural universe in which the truth is continuously evasive: the path of ichthyosarcotoxism, or poisoning by the flesh
of fish. Its most common form, called *ciguatera,* is quite widespread in the
Antilles, in which we measure an annual incidence of thirty-five cases per
100,000 inhabitants[13] with low mortality, unlike the effects of the Japanese *fugu,* the fish of the *takifugu* genus, whose toxin (tetrodotoxin) is
immensely lethal. This group, which remains localized in Asia, belongs
to the large family of tetraodons, notably called *pelpète* or *tchouf-tchouf*
in Creole. To the best of my knowledge, serious poisonings are not reported in the Caribbean, either because the consumption of tetraodons
is avoided (fishing for them is forbidden) or because their effects are less
severe than among the Asian species. Consequently, would it be plausible
that a mastery of this poison might lead to reversible states of catalepsy
where the sorcerer would succeed in awakening the victim? That in no
way explains the further handling and the "reduced life" of the awakened
person, but it is, at any rate, the hypothesis formulated by ethnobiologists
such as Wade Davis, whose experience is narrated here. In the bibliogra-
phy, one feels that Philippe Charlier, at ease in this field from which fo-
rensics is not far away, presents his arguments more solidly on this point,
particularly as Haitian legislation seems inadequate with regard to declaring a person deceased.

Medicine loves to understand, and is not satisfied with mystical explanations, even if it knows that the great mystics and the possessed present some of the most extraordinary symptoms. Psychiatry is not lacking
outrageous cases such as Cotard syndrome, opportunely referred to by

the author, a delirious and suicidal state involving denial of the body and a feeling of immortality. But for Laënnec Hurbon, sociologist and theologian, with whom this account begins, all these attempts at explanation would be too rationalized and implicitly too ethnocentric. In that case, following the example of a successful novelist who imagines the extra-corporeal voyage of an injured person fallen into a coma,[14] a situation that is, in the end, rather analogous to the experience of zombification, we must allow ourselves to wonder, "And what if this were true?" Misery, which leads to despair, gladly leads to gullibility and to mystery, an obstacle over which the spirit of scientific investigation inevitably stumbles. In his preface to the work of journalist and occultist William Seabrook on Haiti[15] cited in Chapter 17, opposite a photo of a Papa Nebo in a white robe, tails, and a top hat, with a skull in one hand and a pickaxe in the other, Paul Morand understood quite well the frustrating limit to consciousness and the impotence of investigating from the outside: "I believe that I know to what extent it is difficult to attend ceremonies other than those that they want to show to foreigners. By definition, everything that is magical is secret." Philippe Charlier, who knows the roots of Vodou well (and from the inside) does not wish to eliminate the mystery, but by embarking with us on this strange and somewhat harrowing trek punctuated by stops in which places and witnesses are questioned, he invites us to imagine what the medical point of view can read beyond the visible.

Alain Froment
Institut de recherche pour le développement
Musée de l'Homme
Département Homme, Nature et Société
Paris, April 2015

NOTES

Chapter 1. Zombie: What Are We Talking About?

1. J. Kerboull, *Le Vaudou. Magie ou religion* (Paris, Robert Laffont, 1973), 137.

Chapter 3. Laënnec Hurbon

1. C. G. Rodero, *Rituales en Haiti* (Madrid, TF Editores, 2001).

2. L. Hurbon, *Les Mystères du vaudou* (Paris, Gallimard, 1993), 87.

3. J.-M. Pelt, *Carnets de voyage d'un botaniste* (Paris, Fayard, 2013).

4. G. E. Berrios, R. Luque, "Cotard's Delusion or Syndrome: A Conceptual History," *Comprehensive Psychiatry* 36 no. 3 (1995): 218.

5. H. Förstl, B. Beats, "Charles Bonnet's Description of Cotard's Delusion and Reduplicative Paramnesia in an Elderly Patient (1788)," *The British Journal of Psychiatry* 160 (1992): 416–418.

6. H. Thomson, "Mindscapes: First Interview with a Dead Man," *New Scientist* 23 (May 2013).

7. L. Hurbon, "Le statut du vodou et l'histoire de l'anthropologie," *Gradhiva* 1 (2005): 53–163.

8. A. Corbet, "Les invisibles omniprésents. Les morts du séisme," in L. Hurbon (dir.), *Catastrophes et environnement. Haïti, séisme du 12 janvier 2010* (Paris, Éd. de l'EHESS, 2014).

Chapter 4. An Overview of Haitian Vodou

1. M. Marcelin, *Mythologie vodou*, Port-au-Prince, Les Éditions haïtiennes, 2 vols., 1949–1950; J. Price-Mars, *Ainsi parla l'oncle* (1928) (Montréal, Leméac, 1973); L. Hurbon, *Dieu dans le vaudou haïtien* (Paris, Payot, 1972); M. Eliade, *Initiation, rites, sociétés secrètes* (Paris, Gallimard, 1959).

2. C. Dauphin, "Rôle et organisation de la musique dans les cérémonies de vaudou," *Bulletin du Bureau national d'ethnologie*, h.s. (2014): 28–43.

3. L. Hurbon, *Les Mystères du vaudou* (Paris, Gallimard, 1993): 13, 33.

4. See Appendix 1 presenting the list of similarities between *loas* and Catholic saints.

5. A. Métraux, *Le Vaudou haïtien* (Paris, Gallimard, 1958).

6. J. R. Descardes, *Dynamique vodou et droits de l'homme en Haïti*, DEA d'études africaines, (Paris, Université Paris I Panthéon-Sorbonne, 1999).

7. J. Kerboull, *Le Vaudou. Magie ou religion* (Paris, Robert Laffont, 1973), 138.

Chapter 6. Max Beauvoir

1. E. W. Davis, *The Serpent and the Rainbow* (New York, Simon & Schuster, 1985).

Chapter 7. Tetrodotoxin

1. C. H. Lee, P. C. Ruben, "Interaction between Voltage-Gated Sodium Channels and the Neurotoxin, Tetrodotoxin," *Channels* 2 no. 6 (2008): 407–412.

2. U. G. Rege, G. H. Tilve, K. G. Nair, "Fresh Fish Poisoning," *Journal of Postgraduate Medicine* 25 no. 2 (1979): 67–69.

3. R. C. Prince, "Tetrodotoxin," *TIBS* 13 (1988): 76–77.

4. M. Asakawa, G. Gomez-Delan, S. Tsuruda *et al.*, "Toxicity Assessment of the Xanthid Crab Demania Cultripes from Cebu Island, Philippines," *Journal of Toxicology* 172367 (2010).

5. C. T. Hanifin, "The Chemical and Evolutionary Ecology of Tetrodotoxin (TTX) Toxicity in Terrestrial Vertebrates," *Marine Drugs* 8 (2010): 577–593.

6. B. L. Williams, "Behavioral and Chemical Ecology of Marine Organisms with Respect to Tetrodotoxin," *Marine Drugs* 8 (2010): 381–398.

7. T. Goto, Y. Kishi, S. Takahashi, Y. Hirata, "Tetrodotoxin," *Tetrahedron* 21 (1965): 2059–2088.

8. See Appendix 2. B. W. Halstead, *Poisonous and Venomous Marine Animals of the World* (Princeton, Darwin Press, 1978: 437–548.

9. C. Y. Kao, "Tetrodotoxin, Saxitoxin and their Significance in the Study of Excitation Phenomena," *Pharmacology Revue* 18 (1966): 997–1049.

10. World Health Organisation (WHO), *Aquatic Marine and Freshwater Biotoxins. Environmental Health Criteria*, Genève, WHO, 1984.

11. A. R. Mills, R. Passmore, "Pelagic Paralysis," *Lancet* 1 (1998): 161–164.

12. S. K. Chew, L. S. Chew, K. W. Wang, P. K. Mah, B. Y. Tan, "Anti-Cholinesterase Drugs in the Treatment of Tetradotoxin Poisoning," *Lancet*, 2 (1984): 108.

13. C.C.P. Silva, M. Zannin, D. S. Rodrigues, *et al.*, "Clinical and Epidemiological Study of 27 Poisoning Caused by Ingesting Puffer Fish (Tetrodontidae) in the States of Santa Catarina and Bahia, Brazil," *Revista do Instituto de Medicina Tropical de São Paulo* 52 no. 1 (2010): 51–55.

14. F. L. Lau, C. K. Wong, S. H. Yip, "Puffer Fish Poisoning," *Journal of Accident and Emergency Medicine* 12 (1995): 214–215.

15. M. Y. Lan, S. L. Lai, S. S. Chen, D. F. Hwang, "Tetrodotoxin Intoxication in a Uraemic Patient," *Journal of Neurology, Neurosurgery, and Psychiatry* 67 (1999): 127–128.

16. P. Tanner, G. Przekwas, R. Clark *et al.*, "Tetrodotoxin Poisoning associated with Eating Puffer Fish Transported from Japan to California," *Morbidity and Mortality Weekly Report (CDC)* 45 no. 19 (1996): 389–491.

17. Y. K. Loke, M. H. Tan, "A Unique Case of Tetrodotoxin Poisoning," *Medical Journal of Malaysia* 52 no. 2 (1997): 172–174.

18. J. Field, "Puffer Fish Poisoning," *Journal of Accident & Emergency Medicine* 15 (1998): 334–336.

19. F. R. Chowdhury, H.A.M. Nazmul Ahasan, A.K.M. Mamunur Rashid, A. Al Mamun, S. M. Khaliduzzaman, "Tetrodotoxin Poisoning: A Clinical Analysis, Role of Neostigmine and Short-Term Outcome of 53 Cases," *Singapore Medical Journal* 48 no. 9 (2007): 830–839.

20. H.A.M. N. Ahasan, A. A. Mamun, S. R. Karim *et al.*, "Paralytic Complications of Puffer Fish (Tetrodotoxin) Poisoning," *Singapore Medical Journal* 45 no. 2 (2004): 73–74.

21. L. Ngy, S. Taniyama, K. Shibano *et al.*, "Distribution of Tetrodotoxin in Pufferfish Collected from Coastal Waters of Sihanouk Ville, Cambodia," *Journal of the Food Hygienic Society of Japan* 5 no. 49 (2008): 361–365.

22. H. L. Yin, H. S. Lin, C. C. Huang *et al.*, "Tetrodotoxication with *Nassauris glans*: A Possibility of Tetrodotoxin Spreading in Marine Products near Pratas Island," *American Journal of Tropical Medicine and Hygiene* 73 no. 5 (2005): 985–990.

23. H. H. Chua, L. P. Chew, "Puffer Fish Poisoning: A Familial Affair," *Medical Journal of Malaysia* 64 no. 2 (2009): 181–182.

24. Y. Nagashima, T. Matsumoto, K. Kadoyama *et al.*, "Tetrodotoxin Poisoning Due to Smooth-Backed Blowfish *Lagocephalus inermis* and Toxicity of *L. inermis* caught off the Kyushu Coast, Japan," *Food Hygiene and Safety Science* 2 no. 53 (2012): 85–90.

25. N. Homaira, M. Rahman, S. P. Luby *et al.*, "Multiple Outbreaks of Puffer Fish Intoxication in Bangladesh, 2008," *American Journal of Tropical Medicine and Hygiene* 83 no. 2 (2010): 440–444.

26. E. W. Davis, "The Ethnobiology of the Haitian Zombi," *Journal of Ethnopharmacology,* 9 (1983): 85–104.

27. E. W. Davis, *The Serpent and the Rainbow* (New York, Simon & Schuster, 1985).

28. E. W. Davis, *The Ethnobiology of the Haitian Zombi,* doctoral thesis, Department of Biology, Harvard University Archives, 1987.

29. W. H. Anderson, "Tetrodotoxin and the zombi phenomenon," *Journal of Ethnopharmacology* 23 (1988): 121–126.

30. C. Benedek, L. Rivier, "Evidence for the Presence of Tetrodotoxin in a Powder Used in Haiti for Zombification," *Toxicon* 27 (1989): 473–480.

31. T. Yasumoto, C. Y. Kao, "Tetrodotoxin and the Haitian Zombie," *Toxicon* 24 (1986): 747–749.

32. E. W. Davis, *The Serpent and the Rainbow* (New York, Simon & Schuster, 1985).

33. G. B. Frank, C. Pinsky, "Tetrodotoxin-Induced Central Nervous System Depression," *British Journal of Pharmacology*, 26 (1966): 435–443.

34. C. B. Berde, U. Athiraman, B. Yahalom *et al.*, "Tetrodotoxin-Bupivacaine-Epinephrine Combinations for Prolonged Local Anesthesia," *Marine Drugs* 9 (2011): 2717–2728.

35. F. R. Nieto, E. J. Cobos, M. A. Tejada *et al.*, "Tetrodotoxin (TTX) as a Therapeutic Agent for Pain," *Marine Drugs* 10 (2012): 281–305.

Chapter 8. My First Zombie

1. J. Ravix, *Temps de certitudes. Journal d'un itinéraire* (Port-au-Prince, Thérad, 2002).

2. J. Ravix, *Place de l'enclouage à foyer fermé dans le traitement des fractures de la diaphyse fémorale*, doctoral thesis in medicine, Université de Besançon, 1974.

Chapter 9. In Erol's Peristyle

1. F. X. Gomez, "Erol Josué, port de prince vaudou," *Libération* April 12, 2013.

2. C. E. Peters, *La Croix contre l'asson* (Port-au-Prince, La Phalange, 1960).

3. B. A. Kesler, "Chant de deuil traditionnel haïtien: enjeux de patrimonialisation," *Bulletin du Bureau national d'ethnologie* h.s. (2014): 133–146.

Chapter 10. On the Tomb of Narcisse . . .

1. M. Beauvoir, *Lapriyè Ginen* (Port-au-Prince, Edisyon Près Nasyonal d'Ayiti, 2008), 13.

Chapter 12. Zombies at the Courthouse

1. E. L. Bell, "The Historical Archaeology of Mortuary Behavior: Coffin Hardware from Uxbridge, Massachusetts," *Historical Archaeology* 24 (1990): 54–78.

2. M. Gilbert, R. Busund, A. Skagseth, P. Nilsen, J. Solbo, "Resuscitation from Accidental Hypothermia of 13.7 °C with Circulatory Arrest," *Lancet* 355 no. 9201 (2000): 375–376.

3. Code pénal haïtien (mis à jour par Jean Vandal), section "Crimes et délits contre les particuliers," (Port-au-Prince, 2007): 59–60.

4. E. Jeanty, "Le statut juridique du *zombi*," *Le Nouvelliste* May 28, 2010.

5. http://www.uramel.org.

Chapter 15. Mireille the *Mambo*

1. R. Bastide, *Les Religions africaines au Brésil* (Paris, Presses universitaires de France, 1995).

Chapter 17. Other Zombies ... Dead or Alive

1. W. Seabrook, *L'Île magique. Les mystères du vaudou* (Paris, J'ai lu, 1971), 120–121.

2. W. Seabrook, *L'Île magique. Les mystères du vaudou* (Paris, J'ai lu, 1971), 122–123.

3. Z. Neale Hurston, *Tell My Horse*, 1938.

4. B. Diederich, *"Zombificateur of a Nation and about Zombis and Zombification,"* Port-au-Prince, Bibliothèque Nationale d'Haïti, 2014.

5. B. Diederich, "On the Nature of Zombi Existence," *Caribbean Review* 12 (1983): 14–17, 43–46.

6. J. Kerboull, *Le Vaudou. Magie ou religion* (Paris, Robert Laffont, 1973), 138–139.

7. J. Kerboull, *Le Vaudou. Magie ou religion* (Paris, Robert Laffont, 1973), 139–144.

8. H. W. Ackerman, "The Ways and Nature of the Zombi," *Journal of American Folklore* 414 no. 104: 466–494.

9. T. Verstynen, B. Voytek, *Do Zombies Dream of Undead Sheep? A Neuroscientific View of the Zombie Brain* (Princeton, Princeton University Press, 2014).

10. R. Littlewood, C. Douyon, "Clinical Findings in Three Cases of Zombification," *Lancet* 350 (1997): 1094–1096.

Chapter 18. *Vévé* Drawings

1. M. Beauvoir, *Lapriyè Ginen* (Port-au-Prince, Edisyon Près Nasyonal d'Ayiti, 2008), 33–34.

2. M. Beauvoir, *Lapriyè Ginen* (Port-au-Prince, Edisyon Près Nasyonal d'Ayiti, 2008), 35–36.

Postface

1. http://www.cameroon-info.net/stories/0,13014,@,douala-rebondissement-avantage-a-la-famille-nformi-le-revenant-remis-a-sa-famille.html

2. Éric de Rosny (dir.), *Justice et Sorcellerie*, colloque international de Yaoundé, mars 2005, Paris/Yaoundé, Katharla/Presses de l'université catholique d'Afrique centrale, 2006.

3. Jean-Yves Le Naour, *Le Soldat inconnu vivant* (Paris, Hachette, 2002).

4. *L'Œuvre de Pierre-Corneille Blessebois*: *Le Rut ou la Pudeur éteinte; Histoire amoureuse de ce temps; Le Zombi du Grand-Pérou*, introduction and bibliographical essay by Guillaume Apollinaire (Paris, Bibliothèque des Curieux, 1921).

5. "We went to mass, and from the church we came back to Marigot where we committed a debauchery that lasted two hours longer than the sun. Most of the main inhabitants were present and whosoever wanted to blend whites and blacks was satisfied without any problems." . . .

6. Ernest Pépin, *L'Homme-au-bâton* (Paris, Gallimard, 1992).

7. J. C. Martínez Cruzado, "El uso del ADN mitochondrial para descubrir las migraciones precolombinas al Caribe: Resultados para Puerto Rico y expectativas para la República Dominicana," *KACIKE: Revista de la Historia y Antropología de los Indígenas del Caribe*, 2002, electronic edition.

8. Half of these white slaves would die before the end of the contract. In 1720, the date when this low-cost system of indentured servitude ends, the price of a "negro with talent" is high, in the range of 2,000 to 3,000 pounds, when the salary of a skilled French worker is only around one pound per day.

9. Certain authors such as Arsène Nganga or Lilas Desquiron (*Racines du vodou*, Port-au-

Prince, Deschamps, 1990) speak in favor of a reevaluation of the Bantu contribution and especially the Kongo contribution of Vodou.

10. Laënnec Hurbon, "Le culte du vaudou. Histoire, pensée, vie," in G. Casalis et al. (dir.), *Croyants hors frontières. Hier, demain* (Paris, Buchet/Chastel, 1975): 225–249.

11. François Makandal or Mackandal, a slave taken in Africa, sentenced to burn at the stake in 1758 for poisonings and witchcraft, suspected of being a Vodou priest, and considered as one of the pioneers of the Haitian Revolution of 1791, although the popular imagination has made Makanda into an off-putting figure.

12. Alfred Métraux, *Le Vaudou haïtien* (Paris, Gallimard, 1958).

13. J.-P. Quod et al., "La ciguatera dans les Dom-Tom: aspects épidémiologiques et physiopathologiques," *Recueil de médecine vétérinaire*, special edition *Mer* (1994): 1–6.

14. Marc Lévy, *Et si c'était vrai?* (Paris, Robert Laffont, 2000).

15. William Buehler Seabrook, *L'Île magique* (Paris, Firmin Didot, 1932).

APPENDIXES

1. Similarities between *loas* of Haitian Vodou and Catholic Saints

Loas	Saints
"Rainbow" Damballa	Moses (*rada* rite)
"The Torch" Damballa	Saint Patrick (*petro* rite)
Tokan Aïda Ouèdo (female notion of Damballa)	Our Lady of the Immaculate Conception or Saint Veronica
Piè (Peter) Damballa and Piè Dantor	Saint Peter
Grann (Grandmother) Alouba or Aloumandia	Saint Anne
Legba Mèt Kafou (Maître Carrefour)	Saint Lazarus
Legba Mèt Pòtay (Maître Portail)	Saint Peter
Atibon Legba	Saint Anthony (the Hermit, *rada* rite; of Padua, *petro* rite)
Simbi dlo (water)	Saint Raphael
Simbi Andeïzo (between two waters)	Saint Andre
Azaka Médé	Saint Isadore the Laborer
Maîtresse Erzulie Fréda Dahomey	Sainte Rose, Virgin Miracle, Mater Dolorosa, Virgin Caridad or Saint Elizabeth
Maîtresse Erzulie Dantor	Our Lady of Czestochowa—Mater Salvatoris, The Black Virgin of Poland, Our Lady of Mount Carmel, Our Lady of Perpetual Help or Our Lady of Altagracia
Maîtresse the Siren	Our Lady of the Assumption
Baron Samedi	Saint Martin of Porres
Guédé Nibo	Saint Gerard of Majella

(*continued*)

Loas	Saints
Baron La Croix	Saint Francis of Assisi
Bossou Trois Cornes	Saint Vincent
Ogou Batallah	Saint Phillip
Ogou Balendjo	Saint James the Greater
Ogou Ferraille and Shango	Saint George
Ogou Badagri	Saint Joseph
Ogou Saint Jean or Jean Dantor	Saint John the Baptist
Agassou Gnenin (Djémé)	Saint Augustine
Mambo Aïzan Vélékété	Jesus Christ during his baptism
Lenglesou	Jesus Christ crucified and bloody on the Cross
Maîtresse Clermesine Clermeil	Saint Claire
Maîtresse Philomise Pierre	Saint Philemon

2. List of clinical symptoms that can be present in a person suffering from acute tetrodotoxin poisoning (TTX)

- Oral and perioral paresthesia (pins-and-needles and tingling)
- Nausea
- Vomiting
- Diarrhea
- Abdominal pains
- Vertigo
- Paleness
- Feeling of discomfort
- Ataxia
- General numbness with floating sensation
- Paresthesia of the extremities preceding paralysis of the lower members and of the extremities
- Change of proprioception (throat and larynx being affected first)
- Dysphagia (trouble with swallowing), even complete aphasia (inability to swallow)
- Dysphonia (trouble with voice)
- Mydriasis (dilatation of the pupils)
- Bradycardia (slowing of the heart rhythm)
- Hypotension (decrease of arterial pressure)
- Hypersalivation
- Hypothermia (decrease of body temperature)
- Excessive sweating
- Asthenia (significant fatigue)
- Cyanosis (bluish coloration) of the extremities and of the lips
- Petechial hemorrhages on the body

ACKNOWLEDGMENTS

This anthropological investigation would not have been possible without the help and the involvement of Anaïs Augias, Max Beauvoir, Nadia Benmoussa, Herlyne Blaise and her family, Louise Carmel-Bijoux, Dr. Anne-Laure Chauveau-Muller, Dr. Louis-Marc Girard, Sylvain Girardeau, Laënnec Hurbon, Sophie Jacqueline, Erol Josué, Stéphane Martin, Christophe Moulherat, Anne-Laure Muller, Zlatko Orlic, Véronique Rabuteau, Dr. Jacques Ravix, Patrick Scott, Jean-Philippe Urbach . . . and the *loas* who were kind to me.

I also thank Claudine Savare, a visitor of the peristyle of Port-au-Prince in the 1970s and my first initiator into Haitian Vodou.

The writing of this investigation concluded under the best possible conditions thanks to Lionel Aupart, Géraldine Varin, and the crew of AF Flight 217.

Finally, thank you to Isabelle, Jules, Paul, and Louis who, through their tenderness, illuminated the sometimes very dark abyss of zombification.

GLOSSARY

angajan. A magical/religious pact between a believer and a *loa*. This pact can be either positive or negative in nature.

asson. A kind of rattle belonging to the *houngan* or the *mambo* consisting of a calabash covered with a net into the mesh of which grains of porcelain or snake vertebra are inserted. It is a royal attribute and a symbol of power. During a Vodou ceremony, the priest can use the *asson* to alter the tempo of the ceremony.

ati. High chief of Haitian Vodou. A respected Vodou leader. In the Fon language, *ati* means "tree" or "forest."

baclou. A little golem that works for his master (Guyana).

bagui. Chamber of secrets that is the inner sanctuary of a Vodou temple, containing altars covered with sacred objects and religious imagery.

bain de chance. A ceremonial lake of mud.

baka. A protective totemic animal. An illness-causing goblin.

banda. A very suggestive dance performed by the *loa* that imitates the act of reproduction.

bizango. A Vodou rite and secret society that is often involved in evildoing.

bokonon. A type of Vodou priest in Benin. He has the ability to predict the future.

bokor. A Vodou priest who practices evil magic or a priest of divination.

bouga. A type of toad.

brasero. A migrant worker.

candomblé. A religion practiced mainly in Brazil by the "people of the saint."

Ceiba pentadra. A tree of the tropical forests of the Caribbean, Latin America, and West Africa.

ciguartera. Poisoning related to the consumption of certain fish.

concombre zombi. Datura stramonium, known by the common names jimsonweed or Devil's snare, used in Haiti as a chief ingredient in the potion vodou priests use to create zombies.

condeur. A driver of souls of the dead.

coup de mort. The soul of a person rendered ill by a potion delivered by a *bokor*.

coup de poudre. Sorcerers use a white powder to zombify their victims.

déchoukaj. A Creole term meaning "uprooting" that is generally used to refer to the political upheaval in Haiti following the exile of dictator Jean-Claude Duvalier on February 7, 1986. It refers directly to the persecution of the Vodou religion.

déssoune (déssouni). A ritual that consists of removing the *loa* that has been consecrated and which is still attached to the head of a deceased person. It is a ritual that exemplifies a rite of passage that the Vodou priest or priestess conducts at death.

dorlis. A supernatural creature from the beliefs of the Quimbois of the French Antilles. It is a spirit that enters houses at night in order to force sexual relations on men and women during their sleep.

eau de chance. A protection against evil spells and potions.

fils-de-saint. A medium prepared to receive a spirit or deity.

Fon. A language spoken in Benin.

fufu (fugu). A puffer fish whose poison can be lethal due to tetrodotoxin.

fugu kimo. The liver of a type of puffer fish (*fugu*).

Ginen. The cosmic community of the spirits of the ancestors. It can also refer to the *loa*, their dwelling place, or their servants.

govi. An earthenware jar that contains *loa* or the ancestors, which serves as a tool to communicate with the *loa*.

guédé. Spirit of the dead.

gwo-bon-anj. One of the two parts of the soul.

hounfor. A Vodou temple.

houngan. A type of Vodou priest or healer who embodies qualities such as goodness, wisdom, and judgment.

hounsi. Initiates to Vodou; an accepted devotee at a *hounfor* or temple.

kapok. The cotton-like fluff obtained from the seed pods of the kapok tree.

lakou. Clusters of homes surrounding a central courtyard. An agricultural or family compound.

loa. Spirits who serve as intermediaries between Bondye ("good God") and humanity.

loas guédé. *Loas* of the dead.

loup-garou. A werewolf; A *bokor*'s assistant.

lwa. Traditional spelling of *loa.*

makaya. A division of Vodou that originated in the Congo region.

makout zaka. Straw gunnysack that is commonly used throughout rural Haiti.

mambo. A female high priest or healer who is analogous to the *houngan.*

mamy-wata. A supernatural creature described as a mermaid-like figure with a woman's upper body and the hindquarters of a fish or snake.

mapiang. An epithet often associated with Erzulie.

mapou. The Hawaiian name for Erzulie.

marassa. Known as the Divine Twins. Although they are children, are older than any other *loa.* *Marassa* is associated with fertility.

matou. Sacred Mayan tree that secures the axis of the world and that the deceased climbs to go from one celestial level to another.

Momordica elaterum. A poisonous plant similar to *Datura stramonium.*

n'âme. The spirit that animates the flesh and which, equally mortal, gives off an energy that is transmitted to the earth at the time of death. It can be an immaterial creature that is either good or evil.

Obeah. A parallel to Vodou in Jamaica.

ouanga (wanga). A talisman that lodges *baka.* It can be used for either good or evil.

péristyle. An open courtyard within a house; a Haitian Vodou temple.

pot de tête. A small covered jar that is made to protect initiates from evil magic.

potomitan. The centerpost of the Vodou temple around which offerings are placed and people dance. It is the nexus between the terrestrial and the supernatural.

poudre (à) zombi. Zombie powder made from the flesh of a puffer fish. It contains tetrodotoxin and is potentially lethal.

prise du mort. A type of evil Vodou ceremony.

renvoie. A special ceremony that is most often performed forty-one days after the great departure of the dead.

roga. A magical object targeting a very specific individual.

roucou (woucou). A powder applied to corpses.

Santeria. A religion practiced mainly in Cuba.

shango cult. A religion practiced mainly in Trinity.

soucounyan. A small flying creature in Guadeloupe that can take on the appearance of a ball of fire.

takifugu. A genus of fish whose toxin (tetrodotoxin) is very lethal.

tap-tap. Literally meaning "quick quick," the "tap-tap" is a brightly decorated minibus that is used as part of a shared-ride system in Haiti.

tchouf-tchouf. Creole word for tetraodon.

ti-bon-ang. One of the two parts of the soul.

ti-bonanj. A life force.

vaudou. Voodoo or Vodou. A syncretic religion practiced primarily in Haiti.

veillée. A Vodou vigil.

vévé. A type of religious symbol or drawing used in Vodou rituals. It is traced on the ground and represents the intersection between the living and the ancestors and the *loas*. Each *loa* has his or her own corresponding *vévé*.

z'étoile. The star of destiny that resides in paradise at a distance from the body.

zombi bouteille. A bottle holding a part of a deceased person's soul that is placed in the bottom of the burial vault.

TRANSLATOR'S AFTERWORD

While changing television stations one Sunday morning circa 1985, I stumbled upon the 1972 film entitled *Children Shouldn't Play with Dead Things*. Bob Clark's "B-movie" zombie film is a cult classic. The story centers on a theatre troupe led by a mean-spirited director named Alan that travel together to a small island for a night of amusement. Unbeknownst both to the director and to his actors, the island had previously served as a burial site for deranged criminals. As midnight arrives, Alan conducts a séance to raise the dead. Although nothing initially happens, it is not long before the dead walk again and rain down vengeance on the unsuspecting intruders. Like George A. Romero's 1968 classic zombie film, *Night of the Living Dead*, Clark's picture encapsulated the public's curiosity for the mysticism of Haitian Vodou. The final product, however, was a film that did little more than concretize existing stereotypes surrounding the relatively unknown religion of Haitian Vodou.

At the dawn of the 21st century, both zombie television series and zombie films and enjoy unrivaled popularity. Internet Movie Database's (IMDB.com) listing of the Highest Rated "zombie" Feature Films/TV Series contains hundreds of entries. Among the most popular television series are *We're Alive* (2009–), *iZombie* (2015–), and *The Walking Dead* (2010–). With its seventh season premiering in October 2016, *The Walking Dead* is arguably the most well-received zombie television series of all time. In addition to successful television series such as those mentioned here, numerous zombie films including *Zombieland* (2009), *Abraham Lincoln vs. Zombies* (2012), and *Pride and Prejudice and Zombies* (2016) continue to illuminate the silver screen. Initially connected to the Haitian and African zombie traditions, in its social form, zombie television series and films play on the viewer's fear of monsters and of the unknown, thus tapping into the collective unconscious that Carl Jung defined in the latter half of the 19th century. Zombie television series and films themselves, however, serve other purposes including "to criticize real-world social ills—such as government ineptitude, bioengineering, slavery, greed and exploitation—while indulging our post-apocalyptic fantasies."[1] These topics remain important in the 21st century. Given the increased social and political tensions worldwide, the viewing public's fascination with the zombie apocalypse has reached unparalleled heights.

Philippe Charlier assumes an entirely different perspective on zombies than the one that the media commonly advances; he is a forensic anthropologist investigating the zombie phenomenon at its source (Haiti). Unmotivated by commercialism or media frenzy, Charlier is first and foremost a scientist trained to observe and to investigate. Interestingly, he is a researcher who has achieved a bit of fame in France, most notably for his 2013 analysis of the mummified heart of Richard the Lionheart, the English monarch who died in 1199 and whose heart was embalmed and buried separately from his body. Following the anthropologist's rule-of-thumb that "Whatever you study, you also change," Charlier enters the field of investigation with few presuppositions or prejudices. In fact, there are relatively few of his own conclusions to be found within the text. Outlining the specific vocabulary used within the Vodou religion, Charlier travels throughout the island of Haiti to meet with individuals who have experienced the zombie phenomenon firsthand. These various personalities include Laënnec Hurbon, Max Beauvoir, Erol Josué, and Mireille Aïn. Hurbon is a sociologist and research director at the CNRS (National Center for Scientific Research). Beauvoir is a *houngan* (Vodou priest) who was originally trained as a biochemist. Josué is a dancer, a recording artist, a Vodou priest, and an expert on the Vodou religion's culture and history. Aïn is a Vodou priestess of French origin. Thus, through local testimonies and his own scientific observations, Charlier combines a perspective and an understanding of "zombiism" and the Vodou religion is distinct. Critics have generally been receptive to Charlier's work in this field. This particular investigation has been featured on several media programs including *TV5Monde* and *France Info*.

As a whole, *Zombies: An Anthropological Investigation of the Living Dead* is part scientific observation, part historical narrative. Equipping himself with little more than the trained eye of a scientist, Charlier seeks to reach the heart of the perception of the "living dead" within Haiti. Initiated with a quotation from Nathan Kline, who, from 1981, brought his research in psychopharmacologic drugs to the study of the zombification in Haiti, Charlier defines "zombiism" by first underscoring its immense popularity in the media before providing a general description of the zombie phenomenon. Prior to tracing the steps of his investigation on the island, the forensic scientist outlines three main types of zombies with which his readers are not likely familiar.

In general, the entire Vodou religion is misrepresented within popular culture, especially in the United States. Readers might well ask themselves why the zombie as we understand it today evolved in this way. A February 19, 2010 article in *The New York Times* entitled "Myths Obscure Voodoo, Source of Comfort in Haiti" appearing less than six weeks after the earthquake that decimated Haiti contained the following relevant assessment:

"The media has reported a lot about voodoo but not much of it very insightful or intelligent," said Diane Winston, a professor of religion and media at the University of Southern California. "Voodoo is one of those flashpoints for Americans because it's exotic, unknown and has strange connotations. It may be a matter of underlying racism because voodoo is African and Caribbean in its origins, or because voodoo seems so different from Christianity that it's the perfect Other." [2]

According to Edward Said, father of the seminal postcolonial theoretical text entitled *Orientalism*, "modern thought and experience have taught us to be sensitive to what is involved in representation, in studying the Other, in racial thinking, in unthinking and uncritical acceptance of authority and authoritative ideas." [3] Said claims that the "Orient" is a fictional construct that is created under an external Occidental optic, which serves as an initially fragmented or marginalized identity. For many Westerners, the word "Vodou" conjures up images of dolls with pins stuck in them used as black magic to inflict pain on someone or to raise the dead (zombies). Popular culture created this type of misrepresentation—an

"Othering"—that does not accurately portray Vodou as it has been historically practiced within Haiti. As a religion, Vodou is "a whole assortment of cultural elements: personal creeds and practices, including an elaborate system of folk medical practices; a system of ethics transmitted across generations [including] proverbs, stories, songs, and folklore . . . [it] is more than belief; it is a way of life."[4]

As Winston and other scholars have shown, there are numerous converging forces—mostly external—that fashioned the 20th century perspective of Vodou that continues to thrive in the 21st century. Three significant external forces, in particular, that combined to forge this image of Vodou included the Roman Catholic Church, William Seabrook's book entitled *The Magic Island* (1929), and the U.S. occupation of Haiti (1915–1934). From the 1860s to the 1940s, the Catholic Church conducted anti-superstition campaigns within Haiti that conveyed the general principle that whereas Catholicism constituted a legitimate religion, Vodou, other the other hand was little more than a cult of pagan heretics. Never before in the Western world had the distinction between religion and cult become clearer. William Seabrook's book entitled *The Magic Island* (1929) became the first popular English-language text to directly address the phenomenon of the "living dead" within Haiti. A bestseller in the United States, it inspired a variety of B-movies in the 1930s and 1940s, including the 1932 horror film *White Zombie*, the first feature-length zombie film. Lastly, as a result of its presence in Haiti, the U.S. Military created a cartoonish image of Vodou that crystalized in the hearts and minds of Americans that would only gained momentum as Americans struggled to recover from the scourge of World War II. In addition to serving as a form of escape from present-day realities, zombiism offered a potential cause of the horrors of the war itself. Instability within the souls of man throughout the Interwar period had resulted in the emergence of a creature that would bring punishment to the soulless. Stroke by stroke, Charlier's brush paints a picture of zombiism that patently differs from the image reinforced both by outsiders and by the media.

The reader might question whether or not a text such as *Zombies: An Anthropological Investigation of the Living Dead*, in fact, has the power to change the overarching popular narrative that states that Vodou itself is evil and that zombies are apocalyptic. The flood of feature-length zombie films scheduled to be released in the near future suggests that the Judeo-Christian mindset is not fully primed to receive alternate explanations of either the essence of Vodou or the true nature of zombiism. In a day-and-age in which every nation of the world claims to be increasingly more conscious of both our cultural similarities and our differences, stemming from a basic survival instinct, we sometimes craft our own, often inaccurate, understandings of ideas that are foreign to us. Thus, the words "religion" and "cult" soon become both muddied and predetermined. This viewpoint reminds me of a conversation that I had with a student in my office several years ago. When I asked her what her favorite course was that semester, she answered that it was her "World Religion" class. "What are you discussing in that course?" I asked. She responded, "We are talking about different religions of the world . . . and cults." When I pressed her to differentiate a cult from a religion, she explained that a cult typically does strange things like "have people drink blood" and its members "gather at compounds" in which they can carry out some of the basic functions of life. Her finished answer was greeted by the perplexed look on my face. She immediately appeared embarrassed, paused, and said, "Oh my God! That sounds like my church!" Indeed. We were living in the "Bible Belt" in a part of the country that had hundreds of churches, many of which were massive complexes that included their own schools, gymnasiums, etc. The individuals who attended these churches spent a tremendous amount of time together carrying out various rituals. They made offerings to their "God." They ate the body and drank the blood of a "lamb" that had been sacrificed to save them. One of the central goals of her World Religion course was to learn to evaluate the diverse religions of the world. By correcting herself, my student had satisfied both one of the most essential learning outcomes of the course and she had set herself on the pathway of understanding.

In similar fashion, Charlier sets his reader on the pathway of understanding. It is a "footprint" or a "track" that leads to a richer appreciation of Vodou culture. Rather than encouraging the reader to demonize a topic that they do not fully understand, this text seeks to redefine the position of zombiism within the Vodou religion while simultaneously repositioning that religion within the spectrum of world religions. There is also a strong notion of social justice contained within this text. Zombified individuals are denied the natural rights of the citizen. Several of Charlier's sources, including Emmanuel Jeanty, an attorney in criminal law, are working hard to have zombies granted legal status within Haiti. This is a concept that might initially escape the comprehension of some of Charlier's readers. How can you grant legal status to the "living dead"? Charlier closes his investigation with the following words: "I will come back." Further study of zombiism within Haiti is indeed necessary.

Notes

1. "The Modern Zombie." Zombie Guide Magazine. http://www.zombie-guide.com/the-modern-zombie/

2. Samuel G. Freedman, "Myths Obscure Voodoo, Source of Comfort in Haiti," *The New York Times* On Religion. February 19, 2010. Online edition. Accessed August 8, 2016.

3. Edward Said. *Orientalism.* (New York: Vintage Books, 2005): 327.

4. Leslie Desmangles. *The Encyclopedia of the Paranormal* (Amherst: Prometheus Books, 1996).

PHILLIPE CHARLIER, a researcher at Raymond Poincaré University Hospital and researcher-teacher at Paris Descartes University who has been christened by the press "the Indiana Jones of the graveyards," is a forensic medical examiner, anatamopathologist, and paleopathologist, specializing in the study of ancient human remains and mummies. His recent work includes a study of the remains of Richard the Lionheart, the fake relics of Joan of Arc, and the presumed head of Henri IV.

RICHARD J. GRAY II is associate professor of French at Ashland University. His fields of research include interdisciplinary approaches to French literary studies, postcolonial studies, and Francophone studies. He is the author of *Francophone African Poetry and Drama: A Cultural History since the 1960s* as well as numerous articles.